EIDETIC IMAGERY AND TYPOLOGICAL METHODS OF INVESTIGATION

T0174034

Founded by C. K. Ogden

The International Library of Psychology

COGNITIVE PSYCHOLOGY
In 21 Volumes

EIDETIC IMAGERY AND TYPOLOGICAL METHODS OF INVESTIGATION

Their Importance for the Psychology of Childhood, the Theory of Education and General Psychology

E R JAENSCH

First published in 1930 by
Routledge

Reprinted in 1999 by
Routledge
2 Park Square, Milton Park, Abingdon, Oxfordshire OX14 4RN

711 Third Avenue, New York, NY 10017

First issued in paperback 2014

Routledge is an imprint of the Taylor and Francis Group, an informa company

Transferred to Digital Printing 2007

© 1930 E R Jaensch
Translated from the German by O A Oeser

British Library Cataloguing in Publication Data
A CIP catalogue record for this book
is available from the British Library

Eidetic Imagery and Typological Methods of Investigation
ISBN-13 978-0-415-20960-1 (hbk)
ISBN-13 978-0-415-75790-4 (pbk)

Cognitive Psychology: 21 Volumes
ISBN 978-0-415-21126-0
The International Library of Psychology: 204 Volumes
ISBN 978-0-415-19132-6

DEDICATED TO

MY BROTHER AND COLLABORATOR

CONTENTS

PART I

PART II

PART III

APPENDIX

PART I

EIDETIC IMAGERY AND TYPOLOGICAL METHODS IN PSYCHOLOGY

THE most important aspect of *Eidetics*—the theory of eidetic or perceptual images (*Anschauungsbilder*)—is that its development represents the first systematic application of typological methods of investigation. If these methods are consistently applied, they will, it seems, throw new light on many departments of our science. The new methods of approach, and the insight they give us, are best studied in the field of eidetic images, in which they originated. It is still occasionally assumed that eidetic imagery has been the exclusive material of our investigations. But in this book we shall have occasion to discuss investigations along other lines as well. Nevertheless, the new methods, and the insight they give us, are best described in the field in which they had their origin. For it is in this field that they have their most important applications, whose possibilities have by no means been exhausted, in spite of many years of labour.

Optical perceptual (or eidetic) images are phenomena that take up an intermediate position between sensations and images. Like ordinary physiological after-images, they are always *seen* in the literal sense. They have this property of necessity and under all conditions, and share it with sensations.

1

In other respects they can also exhibit the properties of images (*Vorstellungen*). In those cases in which the imagination has little influence, they are merely modified after-images, deviating from the norm in a definite way, and when that influence is nearly, or completely zero, we can look upon them as slightly intensified after-images. In the other limiting case, when the influence of the imagination is at its maximum, they are ideas that, like after-images, are projected outward and literally *seen*. Just as there are different shades of orange, which all lie somewhere between pure red and pure yellow, so, too, the slightly intensified after-image and the projected, literally visible, memory image are the limiting cases between which the eidetic images lie. It was found that the point between these extremes at which the phenomenon of eidetic images manifests itself, whether it approximates to, or coincides with one or other pole, depends on the psychophysical constitution. We can therefore make use of a similar symbolic representation, as is usual in colour theories. We may imagine a line drawn between the two 'end-points' red and yellow, so that the various shades of yellow are represented by points on this line. Similarly, we may imagine a line drawn between the 'end-points,' pure physiological after-images, and outwardly projected, literally visible, memory images. The points on this line would then represent different types of eidetic images, sometimes approaching after-images, sometimes memory images. Because of the fluctuations in the personality, however, we cannot assign one definite point to the eidetic image, but must assign to it a finite range within which the phenomenon can fluctuate according to the momentarily operative functional circumstances (experimental conditions), now approaching the one pole, now the other. The localization of the phenomenon on our symbolic line depends in the first place, therefore, on a permanent factor, the constitution of the personality. But since the personality often changes in the course of development, it would be better to say that localization depends on a *relatively permanent, constitutionally determined factor*. In the second place, it depends to a lesser degree on a *momentary, functionally determined factor*. This can be introduced at any moment and depends on the particular circumstances or experimental conditions in which we happen to place the person to be investigated.

It must be especially emphasized that this schema has not been evolved by *a priori* construction : we have been led to it by rigorously empirical procedure. Detailed investigations extending over many years, on an extensive material drawn first from Marburg and later from places all over Germany, have repeatedly shown that the phenomena can be brought into line with this schema. We have only placed it at the beginning of these discussions because it gives the clearest preliminary orientation as to the nature of eidetic images. The description of the empirical investigations and their results will soon fill this abstract schema with the life of concrete particulars.

For the great majority of adults there is an unbridgeable gulf between sensations and images. It has always been known that for a few individuals this is not true. Some people have peculiar 'intermediate experiences' between sensations and images. From the description that such people have given of these experiences, and from the characterization we have just given of eidetic images, we must conclude that their 'experiences' are due to eidetic images. These phenomena, it is true, are rare among average adults. Their existence would, however, not have been doubted so often, and they would have been found to be fairly frequent even in adults, if those scientifically interested in such things had not always made their observations on people whose environment and interests were similar to their own, and therefore directed to abstract pursuits. One should occasionally take one's material from amongst people who are more concretely inclined. Better still, subjects should not always be taken from philosophical class-rooms or psychological institutes, but occasionally from an academy of fine arts, or a group of people with artistic leanings and pursuits, to mention a group that is as widely different from the first as possible.

We have often received enquiries as to the methods by which eidetic imagery can best be discovered, especially among school children. For this reason, and also because tests have occasionally been carried out by unsuitable methods, we shall give a few methodical instructions, as far as our limited space allows.

First of all we have to take care that the individuals to be investigated understand us correctly when we talk about phenomena that can literally be *seen*. Otherwise children might understand us to be referring merely to visual *memory images*. We must therefore demonstrate to them exactly what it means to *see* something, although no object is actually present. This will have to be done for some case that is realizable whether the subject has eidetic images or not. The only case where this is possible is in physiological after-images, which are obtained when a simple object of intense colour is fixated for some time. We therefore begin each investigation by showing the subject some after-images. A homogeneous red square (5 cm.²) is placed on a homogeneous gray background and fixated for 20 seconds. When it is taken away, the after-image will generally appear on the gray background. The after-image is generally correctly described in the complementary (or nearly complementary) colour, and this gives us a proof that the statements are correct and based on a real experience. If necessary, the time of fixation can be extended. We then explain to the child in words adapted to its intellectual standard, that something is *seen* here, although there is no object on the gray screen, and that henceforth, whenever we speak of ' seeing,' we mean the sort of seeing that has just been realized in the case of after-images. Something must therefore be seen on the screen ; it must not remain blank as before the experiment. Eidetic images proper, which we wish to bring forth, are usually best seen on a homogeneous dark gray (not black) background of 50° white and 310° cloth-black on the colour disc. We therefore use such a screen from the very beginning, as well as in the later experiments.

After this first experiment, which is merely meant as a preliminary step towards correct understanding of what we require, it is advisable to repeat it—allowing sufficient time to elapse for the first after-image to die away completely—and to determine the duration or the periodic times of the after-image.

This will already single out some of the eidetic cases, namely those in whose eidetic images there is a strong component related to after-images. In these cases the after-image is of longer duration and is generally continuous, instead of vanishing periodically and appearing again for a shorter time. For mass investigations we can therefore begin by presenting some object that is suitable for generating after-images to a whole class, or to the group to be investigated. Those who have intensified after-images can then be singled out for more detailed individual investigation, which is necessary in *every* case. Here we pay special attention to those whose after-images are not in the complementary, but in the original colour, as this points to a relatively high degree of eidetic faculty.

The cases of eidetic imagery that are related to the A.I., and that reveal themselves at this preliminary test, are verified by a second test. A complicated object, *e.g.* a silhouette picture with numerous details,[1] is *fixated* for 15 seconds. When the picture is removed, a non-eidetic will see at most a few details on the screen, as experience has shown. If the subject sees the whole picture, or the majority of the details sharply defined, this points with even greater certainty to the presence of the eidetic faculty. If the colour of this 'after-image' corresponds to that of the original, we have a certain proof. It must always be remembered, however, that in this way we only discover those cases that have a strong A.I.-like component. The clearness of the image is dependent upon rigid *fixation*, just as in A.Is. The other component, which in the majority of cases is also present, is within wide limits independent of previous rigid fixation. In fact it appears more easily after a general inspection, which enables one to become more conscious of the details of an object, and this is an important factor in the conceptual component of E.Is.

The third test is based on this. After a sufficiently long interval, the coloured square that was used in the first test is presented for non-fixating inspection for a shorter time (10-15 secs.). If this results in a picture with sharp contours,

---

[1] The *Münchener Bilderbogen* " Was alles am Morgen geschieht " (published by Braun und Schneider, Munich) has proved to be very suitable. It naturally has to be cut up and only one of the pictures presented at a time. These should not be much larger than a post card for all average cases.

not merely in an irregular blot, we may look upon this as indicating even more conclusively the presence of the eidetic faculty, particularly if the colour is pronounced as well. We may be absolutely certain, if the colour of the image is the same as that of the original square. But we must not content ourselves with a negative result from such a simple object. The test must always be succeeded by one on a complex, interesting picture that has some meaning (*e.g.* represents some scene), because the appearance of the conceptual component is not so dependent on fixation or on factors that influence the sense organ. It depends rather on the interest taken in the picture and on the involuntary attention, which is aroused by this interest. The scenic silhouettes, which have been used above, are best used again, because of the strong impression they make on the involuntary attention. Moreover, they are very suitable, because one always has to take account of the A.I.-like component. This is present in the majority of cases and demands an intense sense impression, which the silhouettes are able to give. For the other component, which is dependent more on interest, one should always have a fairly large collection of pictures on different subjects at hand, because those cases in which this component is predominant show a very strong selective tendency. Certain types of objects are preferred, and sometimes give rise to clearer E.Is. by themselves, quite independently of the purely optical qualities, and particularly of the sensory intensity of the picture. Thus we have several times found a higher percentage of eidetics among younger children when animal pictures were used, which interested them, than when the to them more uninteresting pictures of houses were used. It must also be noted that the parts of a picture must not be too much alike, as, *e.g.* in the well-known Dieffenbach post cards, since this often prevents the correct reappearance of the particulars in the E.I. Furthermore, there must be an inner connection between the various parts of a picture ; it must have a meaning as a whole, to be appropriate to the laws of imagination, which are obeyed by the conceptual component of many E.Is. In a demonstration during a lecture, a youth, who normally had very pronounced E.Is., was to his own surprise able to see only a few details, and these indistinctly. The reason was that having no pictures he had not seen before, we had made a new one by cutting parts out of the other pictures and sticking them together. In this way we had produced a test-object with no inner coherence.[1]

As a rule the E.Is. are best seen on a dark gray background of the type mentioned above. If the result is negative, however, one should also try the experiment when head and background are in deep shadow, *e.g.* thrown by a piece of cloth, or let the subject try with his eyes closed. It sometimes happens that the E.I. is only visible under these conditions. In the latter case one should particularly note whether there is any colour contrast along the edges. One also finds that in rare cases the E.I. is best seen on a light background. Finally, one should always note whether E.Is. occur spontaneously under special circumstances, particularly in emotionally toned situations. Even in the weak cases that have the conceptual component, such occasional, spontaneous images are hardly ever entirely lacking, since emotional participation is an important factor in this component.

When analysing the nature of E.Is. one should only take

---

[1] In an article by Schwab (*Psychol. Forschung*, Vol. V, 1924), to be discussed later, several pictures are mentioned, but the one reproduced on p. 236 is contrary to almost all the demands that have to be made of a suitable test-object.

into consideration definite, or 'manifest' cases. For a statistical survey, which may follow this analysis, it is necessary also to take into account the 'latent' cases. By 'latent' we understand those cases in which E.Is. are not directly demonstrable, but only indirectly through abnormal properties of A.Is. or memory images.

Although the disposition for E.Is., even in their more pronounced forms, is widely prevalent up to puberty, we must not expect to find the same, or even approximately the same percentage of eidetics everywhere. In this respect the greatest differences exist between one locality and the next, and in the same place between different classes in a school. The eidetic disposition is correlated with certain constitutional types, whose distribution varies from locality to locality, and this explains the variation in the frequency of pronounced eidetic cases. Far more fundamental, apparently, is its dependence on the type of education, in particular on the difference between the so-called *Lernschule* in the old sense and the *Arbeitsschule* in the new. The latter takes far more account of the idiosyncrasies of the child, in particular its natural attention to the world of the senses. This type of school, by continually reinforcing abstract thought with concrete particulars ('object lessons'), takes into account the desire of the child for activity, and in so doing combats 'school passivity' and the lowering of intellectual activity, which otherwise manifest themselves soon after the child's entrance into school. This is probably the reason why statistical enquiries in schools of this type, in many different German towns, have hitherto always yielded an incomparably larger percentage of eidetics than others (H. Freiling). This dependence on the type of education appears to be more fundamental than the dependence

B

on locality. In numerous classes of this kind almost all pupils (85-90 per cent) were eidetics. Moreover, they were all of the strongly developed type, or at least of a medium type. The weaker cases were practically absent. This fact shows most clearly that the eidetic disposition is a normal quality of youth, which is generally prevalent wherever the common antagonistic processes are absent, where, on the contrary, we carefully avoid forcing the youthful mind prematurely into the mould of the adult.[1] This also indicates the pedagogic importance of this disposition.

There is no contradiction between these facts and dependence on the *constitution*, which was mentioned above. For children that grow up under these conditions are not only different in respect of educational aims ; they also show characteristics connected with the eidetic constitution, which are in no way intended by their particular education. Indeed, they are not even known to the teacher. In the case of such children we have to postulate a youthful organization that is determined by these influences, or rather, preserved and guarded by them. Furthermore, the connection between eidetic disposition and general constitutional structure has to be acknowledged, because these favourable conditions are not usually present. Those individuals will therefore prove to be eidetics of the more pronounced type, whose constitution is most favourable to this mode of experience and gives rise to eidetic phenomena in spite of the resisting factors that are usually present.

It must seem exceedingly strange to anyone who has worked with these phenomena, and has been forcibly impressed by the observed facts, that doubts are still occasionally

---

[1] Cf. the monograph of H. Freiling, *Über die psychologischen Grundlagen der Arbeitsschule* (in preparation).

expressed as to the psychic reality of these phenomena, or that some people cannot bring themselves to recognize them as a peculiar, distinct class of psychic phenomena, allocating them instead either to physiological A.Is. or to visual memory images. Anyone who has performed such experiments over and again and on continually fresh material, can never hold this opinion. In many cases an explanation by means of visual memory images is excluded by the accuracy with which pictures are described in every detail. But above all, such an interpretation becomes quite impossible if we consider the way in which such pictures arise and disappear, and the whole attitude of the subjects towards them. The preceding experiment with A.Is. serves to make the difference between mere 'imagining' and actual 'seeing' so clear to moderately intelligent children, that the possibility of confusion is excluded. With eidetic adults, who are not at all rare, and who are always used as controls, such confusion is naturally impossible. The difference between actually seeing and merely imagining is particularly clear when the E.I. develops gradually, or when it vanishes gradually. " Now I see this . . .", " Now that . . . is beginning to appear," children will say, pointing to a particular spot on the screen. " I know that . . . was also there, but I do not *see* it." " Ah! now I see it!" " Now that . . . is disappearing." " Now it is coming back." Very often the E.I. is richer than the memory image. Questions about certain particulars can at first not be answered. But when the E.I., which often only develops gradually, has become clear in all its details, these questions can be answered. It is very impressive to watch how an inscription in the picture, *e.g.* a placard, cannot at first be remembered, and how a letter appears now here, now there, until the whole writing can be deciphered. Phenomena such as these have time and again convinced the most sceptical, whenever they were demonstrated, here and elsewhere, on school children that were complete strangers to us. Just as convincing for even the most unbelieving spectator are cases that at first look as though they are going to be failures. During a lecture with demonstrations, which I delivered in Magdeburg, for instance, the boy at first declared most emphatically that he " could not see it distinctly." When the curtains over the windows had been drawn apart, so that more light fell on the screen, he suddenly called out, " Now it is quite distinct," and at once began to give a description of the picture in minute detail.

No one will doubt that A.Is. can literally be seen, and we can always verify the correctness of a statement by the colour. The same applies to those E.Is. that appear in the complementary colours of the original picture. In their behaviour, and particularly in colouring, they resemble A.Is. in many respects. But there is an intimate relation between E.Is. in the natural colours of the original, and those resembling A.Is., which are in complementary colours. For most subjects who were able to produce E.Is. in the original colours when the object was interesting and full of detail, had only complementary, A.I.-like E.Is. when an object was used that was poor in detail, homogeneous, or uninteresting (e.g. a homogeneous coloured square). Now the attitude of the subjects, their method of description, etc., is the same in both cases. Indeed, it may happen that in one and the same picture a part that is interesting and rich in detail appears in the original colours, while a part poor in detail appears in complementary colours. There is a constitutional type that is susceptible to treatment with calcium (see below). In pronounced cases of this type all E.Is., as well as A.Is., appear only in the original colours. When the calcium treatment has taken effect, and the eidetic disposition has become weaker, these phenomena begin to manifest themselves in complementary colours, so that negative A.Is., which were unobtainable by any method before, now appear for the first time. Conversely, a latent eidetic disposition in a subject of this type can occasionally be roused to the highest degree by treatment with potassium, which physiologically has the opposite effect to calcium, but only while the potassium is effective.[1]

To admit all this, but because of these relations to classify E.Is. as being the same as A.Is., would be to overlook all the essential properties that distinguish them from A.Is. and that cause them to obey, to a greater or less degree, not only the laws of A.Is. but those of visual imagery. In particular, it would mean disregarding their frequent manifestation of the original colours and the fact that, unlike A.Is., which are always two-dimensional, they can be three-dimensional like a three-dimensional test-object—and once more let it be emphasized that they are in every case *literally seen*. For details we must refer the reader to the special investigations. We shall mention one more example, which perhaps demonstrates most clearly the relation of E.Is. to M.Is., and, on the other hand, the differences between them. It also shows the relation of even the strongest E.Is. to A.Is., by means of which we are always particularly well able to check the statements of our subjects. It is the case of ' memory after-images ' (*Vorstellungsnachbilder*), which only occur in children who have the eidetic faculty very strongly developed. There is, however, no doubt at all about their occurrence in such subjects. If strongly eidetic children, who have never

[1] Walther Jaensch, *Münchener Medizinische Wochenschrift*, 1922.

been used in experiments on A.Is. and do not know their colours, are requested to *imagine* vividly a coloured object, *e.g.* a red square, without actually being shown such an object, then this object can appear on the homogeneous gray screen in front of the subject in its complementary colour when the subject opens his eyes. We mention this particular example, because it once more justifies from a new angle the representation used at the beginning, in which memory images and after-images were represented as end-points of a line containing eidetic images, thus presupposing a relation between memory image and after-image phenomena, which are so often regarded as having no connection.[1]

But the most conclusive and most general proof that E.Is. are literally *seen*, is that E.Is. are within wide limits subject to the same laws as sensations and perceptions. Our subjects do not know anything about these laws, and the fact that they are obeyed cannot therefore be the result of suggestion. All the researches on the parallel behaviour of E.Is. and sensations or perceptions—and they have been repeated at great length, with many variations, and on continually fresh material—are so many control-experiments and proofs for the reality of these phenomena,[2] as well as for the impossibility of simply classifying them either as A.Is. or as M.Is. These proofs have, for instance, been given by experiments on the so-called Horopter deviation, the co-variant phenomenon, the

[1] This fact has also to be kept in mind with respect to the doubts that are expressed against our conception of A.Is., E.Is., and M.Is., as a series of ' memory levels,' which links A.Is. and E.Is. Dr Freiling drew my attention to the fact that W. Wundt, whom P. Petersen (*W. Wundt und seine Zeit.* Frommanns Klassiker der Philosophie, XIII, Stuttgart, 1925) now includes under our ' permanent eidetics,' seems to have had memory after-images (acc. to Ch. Féré, *Rev. philosophique*, 20, 1885. P. 364).

[2] Cf. E. R. Jaensch, *Über den Aufbau der Wahrnehmungswelt*, Leipzig, 1923, 2nd edition, 1927, and *Über Grundfragen der Farbenpsychologie*, Leipzig, 1930.

Aubert phenomenon, the Purkinje phenomenon [1] (in particular with E.Is. in complementary colours, but also with E.Is. in natural colours, though less conclusively), in the phenomena of colour transformation and in other colour phenomena. Further, we were able to show that *in pronounced cases the perceptions of real objects also showed properties, deviating from the properties of normal perceptions, that obeyed the same structural laws as E.Is.* The perceptions during the eidetic phase demonstrate very clearly the close relation of E.Is. to the processes of perception. The E.Is. must, therefore, be separated from A.Is. and M.Is.

Although E.Is. in all pronounced cases are very distinct, they are not in general confused with real objects. In the

---

[1] According to the ' duplicity theory,' which is widely accepted and well-founded, the Purkinje phenomenon is connected with the fact that different receptors are active in our eye during daylight and twilight vision, the cones in the former, the rods in the latter. (v. Kries, cf. G. E. Müller, *Darstellung und Erklärung der verschiedenen Typen der Farbenblindheit,* Göttingen, 1924.) One may perhaps be inclined to argue that as there is no sensory stimulus in E.Is., different receptor organs cannot be involved, wherefore the condition for the manifestation of the Purkinje phenomenon is absent. This fact seems to speak all the more strongly against what was mentioned above, since, according to other circumstances, which cannot be discussed here, an explanation by means of experience or associations is hardly feasible. But to argue thus would be to overlook that the psychophysical personality, for the purposes of psychology, physiology, inner medicine, and neurology, is more and more being proved to be a system of ' levels,' in whose various levels the same function can be represented in modified forms. We have an example here in different memory levels (A.I., E.I., M.I.). It can be compared with others : the equivalence of the result of certain ionic displacements in the bodily fluids and excitatory impulses in the vegetative nervous system (F. Kraus and his school) ; the peripheral and at the same time central representation of certain metabolic processes, which manifest themselves, *e.g.* in the fact that tetany and diabetes can be caused simultaneously peripherally and centrally ; the relatively peripherally and at the same time centrally represented processes of colour vision that are manifest in colour blindness, which can be caused by ' outer ' or ' inner ' factors (colour theory of G. E. Müller and the, in this respect, similar ' zonal ' theory of v. Kries), etc. From our experiments we shall also have to assume a relatively central and a relatively peripheral representation in the Purkinje phenomenon.

majority of cases, they merely have the character of *pictures*, which, nevertheless, are seen in the literal, optical sense. They may therefore be compared to the pictures produced by a magic lantern. It must be added, though, that solid objects are not necessarily always seen two-dimensionally in the E.I. Very often they are seen three-dimensionally. Often, too, the colours of the E.I. are more pronounced, ' brighter,' or more ' glowing,' than those of the test-object.

Apparently there has occasionally been some confusion, because attempts have been made to incorporate E.Is. into the well-known schema of Jaspers :

Perception.	*Imagination.*
Perceptions are ' bodily '	Images are ' pictorial '
(they have an objective	(they have a subjective
character).	character).

As a matter of fact, the majority of eidetic phenomena cannot be placed in this schema. But that is no proof against their psychic reality ; it is merely a proof that the schema of Jaspers [1] is neither valid nor exhaustive. It has not been obtained by strictly empirical, psychological methods, but probably from *a priori* considerations, or by abstraction from the everyday experience of normal psychology, even if it is subsequently applied to the empirically given diseased material. Although the word ' pictorial ' appears in the schema, pictorial phenomena in the true sense of the word, as *e.g.* lantern projections or A.Is., are missing. These have in all respects perceptual properties, but can at the same time be distinguished from real objects, and are therefore not ' bodily ' in the sense of Jaspers. I believe that the mis-

[1] Jaspers, *Allgemeine Psychopathologie*, 2nd edition, Berlin, 1920.

understanding, which leads to the confusion of E.Is. with vivid M.Is., is due to the deserved popularity of Jaspers' book and to the circumstance that the schema contained in it only takes account of that special form of pictorialness manifested by M.Is., apart from the ' bodily ' properties of perceptual objects regarded as objective and real. But this leaves out of account pictorial quality in the true sense of the word, *i.e.* the pictorial quality that is literally presented to perception through sensory optical processes. Now that is characteristic of the majority of eidetic phenomena. Therefore these phenomena will always puzzle those who believe that they can be brought under the Jaspers schema. But the schema is imperfect precisely in the point that is of essential importance here. Several observations I have made, particularly during discussions with psychiatrists, have induced me to emphasize this misunderstanding. The work of Schwab,[1] who uses the concepts of Jaspers throughout, is fundamentally influenced by this misunderstanding.

[1] G. Schwab, " Vorläufige Mitteilung über Untersuchungen zum Wesen der subjektiven Anschauungsbilder," *Psychol. Forschung*, Vol. V, 1924. Thanks to the loyal co-operation of Professor Gruhle, two of my collaborators, my brother and Dr Freiling, had an opportunity of examining the Heidelberg material used by Schwab in his investigations. It was proved beyond question that these cases were not eidetic at all, and it is therefore plain that the author only met with A.Is. and M.Is. It was also in accord with our own experience that such non-eidetics, or at most ' latent ' eidetics, very often make no sharp distinction between actual seeing and mere imagining. This is quite understandable, since they do not know E.Is., which can be seen, but only know M.Is. Real, ' manifest ' eidetics on the other hand, do make a sharp distinction between the two, as we have found over and over again, particularly after we have made clear to them, by means of A.Is., what we mean by an optically real image.

Schwab mentions his subject 10 as an example of an observer who really sees something. But from the records in question we can, in fact, find no evidence for anything but ordinary A.Is. Naturally we, too, would look upon observers of this type, of whom we also know large numbers, as useless for eidetic investigations. A more careful analysis with more accurate

In exceptionally strong cases, particularly in the strictly 'unitary cases' to be discussed presently, E.Is. and real objects can, under certain conditions, be confused with one another. According to extensive and varied experiments this is especially the case when the objects are of a *simple* kind, *e.g.* threads or coloured squares, and when care is taken that E.Is. of similar objects are seen amongst the real objects.[1] *But even in the more pronounced cases, particularly among children, in which such confusions do not generally occur, there is still an intimate connection between the structure of perceptions and that of E.Is., so that both classes of phenomena obey similar*

methods than were possible here on account of the limited time might possibly have discovered traces of a *latent* eidetic disposition. But there certainly was not a single *manifest* eidetic present, and it is these alone that can be used to analyse the nature of subjective E.Is. To start from rudimentary and doubtful cases, instead of from manifest ones, in order to arrive at a conception of the whole complex of phenomena, would be like the procedure of a historian who tries to reconstruct some event from very imperfect and meagre sources, when complete and reliable ones are at his disposal. As a matter of fact my collaborators found very well developed eidetic cases in Heidelberg schools.

The test picture published by Schwab (p. 336), which was used together with others that are only mentioned in the text, fails to conform to almost every condition for a satisfactory test-object. It lacks (1) a sensible coherence ; (2) it contains a large number of similar or approximately similar elements ; (3) there are a number of regions of the same colour and shape sometimes symmetrically arranged. Now ' spatial transformation ' is common in E.Is., and these factors represent conditions that, as it were, challenge ' spatial transformation,' that is, incorrect reproduction, to take place (cf. E. R. Jaensch, *Über den Aufbau der Wahrnehmungswelt*, pp. 155 *et seq.*, "Über Raumverlagerung," etc.). The article of Schwab cannot therefore be regarded as a contribution to the nature of E.Is.

M. Zillig in her first re-examination of the eidetic investigations in Würzburg (*Fortschritte d. Psychol.*, edited by Karl Marbe, Vol. V, 1922), and particularly H. Zeman of the Viennese institute in a recent article (*Zeitschr. f. Psychol.*, 96, 1924), both report on work that was carried out with exemplary thoroughness and objectivity and arrived at results that are in very good accord with our own, except for local differences.

[1] H. Bamberger, " *Über das Zustandekommen des Wirklichkeitseindrucks der Wahrnehmungswelt*," 16 *Ergänzungsbd. Zeitschr. f. Psychol.*, 1930.

laws, which in the limiting cases are identical.[1] Thus we find, *e.g.* that simple objects like threads, which in reality are fixed, move when the gaze or the attention wander in a similar, or in the same way in which the E.Is. move *in the majority of cases* when such movements of gaze or attention are executed. Under the influence of these functional processes the construction of the perceptual world gradually takes place, and the space-values of the retina become fixed, particularly those space-values that are the basis of ' transverse retinal disparity ' or ' binocular parallax,' which is the centre of theories of spatial perception. We speak of transverse disparity, when one and the same object throws images on the two eyes that differ in the horizontal direction. In general this will be the case when an object also extends away from the eyes of an observer, *i.e.* when it has depth. A line AB, lying in the plane of sight of an observer, but extending away from him at an angle, will in general appear under different visual angles at the two eyes, and will therefore give rise to ' transversely disparate ' images on the retina. This disparity, which is the surest and most compelling criterion of depth for the adult, is by no means the only determining factor for the perception of depth in the early phase of vision ; indeed, it does not even determine depth with approximate certainty, neither as regards direction (*i.e.* whether it is situated in front or behind) nor as regards magnitude. This has been proved by detailed investigations of an extensive material consisting of children who had a strong eidetic disposition, and particularly of children that

---

[1] This special structure of the perceptions, which follows the laws of E.Is., is therefore *of common occurrence in youth.* It is by no means limited to the ' strictly unitary cases ' mentioned above, in which E.Is. are confused with real objects. The two cases must be sharply distinguished : the latter is very much rarer, whilst the former is widely prevalent.

belong to the 'unitary type' or are close to it (cf. Ella Mayer, *Die Funktionsschichten der räumlichen Wahrnehmung. Ph.D. thesis, Marburg, 1924*). Optical localization and the spatial structure of the perceptual world are here seen to be dependent on optically dynamic processes and above all by images that are projected outward and become visible in the literal sense of the term. In the early phases of vision this is always the case.[1] It is during this phase, for instance, that the 'approximate constancy in size of optical objects' develops, in a way that can be traced experimentally. By this term we mean the well-known fact that within certain limits objects that are increasing their distance from us seem to remain approximately of the same size, or at any rate do not diminish as rapidly as the retinal image, which diminishes in exact proportion to the distance. For our knowledge and our memory, objects have a *constant* size. This conceived, constant size to a large extent also determines perceived size during this early phase, in which vision is determined in the widest degree by the M.Is. that are projected outward and become visible.

v. Kries had already emphasized the relation between the structure of spatial perceptions and spatial concepts. He considered the relation to be so intimate, that he proposed speaking only of '*Raumvorstellung*.' In connection with this, v. Kries renewed Kant's philosophical criticism, as A. Riehl had done before along similar lines, according to which our picture of the world is produced by the fitting of sensory

[1] We wish to emphasize particularly the extraordinarily wide distribution of this type of structure of the perceptual processes in very young children, because of certain doubts expressed by Gordon W. Allport ("Eidetic Imagery," *Brit. Journ. Psych.*, XV, 1924). Although he accepts eidetic phenomena as facts, he doubts the validity of our view that the structure of the original perceptions is related to that of E.Is.

contents into a conceptual schema that reduces them to order. So this at least is true of Kant's view, that an essential part of the form in which our perceptual contents are given originates in the mental sphere. The facts we have mentioned, and the possibility of tracing them further, provide the basis for bringing to light the central and justifiable core of these historically most important doctrines, by taking into account the demands made by our rigorously empirical way of thinking. It is this very structure of the mental sphere, which dominates our perceptions, that provided the starting-point for the efforts of v. Kries and others to renew the Kantian criticism—in so far as these attempts took account of the theory of perception at all.

This relationship of perceptual and conceptual nature is explained by the proof that perceptions and memory images are developed from an ' undifferentiated unity ' of both, which is neither perception nor ideation—as these are found in the fully developed, non-eidetic adult. It combines the traits of both classes of phenomena in itself ; for it is either a direct eidetic image, or approximates in its behaviour to E.Is. Various stages of this phase of development can be demonstrated in children. Its purest form is evident in those extreme ' unitary cases ' in which, as was mentioned before, there is as yet no pronounced differentiation between E.Is. and perceptions, since both can be confused with each other under certain conditions. This phase of development is still in evidence to a greater or lesser degree in those cases where perceptions conform more or less to the laws of E.Is.[1] It is

[1] It is still occasionally overlooked that this peculiar nature of *perceptual processes* during the eidetic phase of development is the factual basis of the *theory of perception* developed by us. We must emphasize this in view of the recent publication by Gordon W. Allport (" Eidetic Imagery," *Brit. Journ. Psych.*, Vol. XV, October 1924). He admits the reality of eidetic

no proof to the contrary that this phase cannot be demonstrated in each individual life period, and therefore not in
every child. In such cases the process of differentiation
between the sphere of perception and the sphere of ideas has
taken place in previous generations, so that the individual
is born with a comparatively ready-made and well-differen-
tiated perceptual function. Many remarkable and surprising
statements made by explorers can be explained in the simplest
way, if we assume that the eidetic disposition is on the
average far more widely prevalent in primitive civilizations,

phenomena, but is not willing to support their application to theories about
the development of *perceptions*.

The occurrence of the ' unitary type,' in whom perceptions are subject
to laws that are more or less similar, or, in limiting cases exactly equal, to
those of E.Is., is not a *theory* or *hypothesis*, but an empirically proven *fact·*
Later investigations, in which younger children have been used to a greater
extent, confirmed this anew (cf. the remarks made above on ' transverse
disparity '). But it has already been made thoroughly certain by the
material published in the monograph " *Über den Aufbau der Wahrnehmungswelt* " (Leipzig, 1923, Joh. Ambr. Barth). Allport does not mention
this peculiarity of perceptions, which is also widely prevalent in children,
nor does he mention our monograph in his index. He does mention,
however, a general review by Koffka, which appeared shortly after our
very first publications. That Koffka's premature criticism is entirely beside
the point, must be clear to any reader of our monograph.

Allport's objection, that the eidetic unitary phase should be demonstrable
in all children, can be met by the consideration that the processes con-
tributing to the development of space-perception, which we have found
in a large percentage of cases, may have been completed in previous
generations. The ' space-values ' would then be an innate disposition
in the individual. Even A. Bielschowsky, one of the most determined
protagonists of the theory of innate space-values, as I know from con-
versations with him, only assumes this ' innateness ' for the individual
life. Within the ascendancy he allows or presupposes a gradual *development*
of the space-values.

There may, of course, be differences due to race even here. We pre-
sumably find even on these elementary levels of mental life similar conditions
to those postulated by my neo-philological colleagues, Deutschbein and
Wechssler, for the higher levels : that the German stands between the
Anglo-American and the Romance race in his subjective behaviour. We
shall bring forward more exact facts for this in another place. Here we
shall merely mention that a colleague from a Spanish university

even among adults, and that in particular a much closer relation between E.Is. and perceptions exists for them.[1]

The proof that these developmental processes take place within the individual also throws new and suggestive light on the *development of the organ of sight* in man and the vertebrates (cf. *Über den Aufbau der Wahrnehmungswelt*, ch. xiii). These remarks should suffice to indicate how important the study of the eidetic phase of development is for the construction of our perceptual world.[2]

But the relations that have been discovered between the eidetic phase of development and the structure of our perceptual world are not only of importance to questions of general philosophy. They are, it seems to us, of immediate and great importance to pedagogy. The value that is placed on pedagogical work, the emphasis that is given it, and the hopes that are centred in it, are always measured by the degree of *plasticity* or educability that the psychic organization is estimated to possess. It has always been

(Professor A. Encinas, Santander), visited us last year in order to be introduced to eidetics, because he hoped that it would provide some clue to phenomena that are being talked about a great deal in Spain at the moment. Hundreds of sworn statements have been made to the effect that certain pictures of saints perform miracles, step out of their panels, carry out actions, etc. These assertions are based in particular on sworn statements by scientifically educated persons, like engineers, doctors, etc., who are accustomed to sober thinking. We demonstrated the peculiarities of perceptive processes in eidetic subjects to our Spanish colleague. What he saw strengthened his supposition that these peculiarities were the key to the phenomena in Spain (cf. the remarks below as to the great psycho-physiological differences within the relatively small territory of the province Hessen-Nassau).

[1] The ethnologist R. Thurnwald, who has lived amongst primitive peoples for a long time, has undertaken to direct the attention of those of his colleagues, who are returning to primitive peoples, to this subject. We have been perfectly conscious that there has been a gap here, as Allport pointed out, and we had particularly emphasized this in our monograph.

[2] For more details, the reader is referred to the monograph.

correctly supposed that the higher psychic events can be influenced with ease, but the more elementary ones only with difficulty. But it was presupposed that this 'plastic' nature of the psychic only began above the perceptual sphere, which was almost always regarded as something absolutely rigid and merely physiologically determined. The new results about the structure of perceptions show the range within which human nature is ' plastic ' to be far wider than even the most optimistic were willing to admit. They show that even the perceptual sphere is plastic, although it has always been regarded as being the most rigid and least plastic part of the mind's inventory—as, indeed, it is. All this is not theory, but experimentally discovered fact.

Primitive organisms can always respond to environmental influences with the same reactions as their ancestors, since these influences remain to a very wide extent constant for them. But for higher organisms, particularly for man, the change in environmental conditions that arises in the course of generations, becomes an important factor. Now in the higher organisms, and particularly in man, the majority of reactions does not follow immediately on stimuli from the environment, but on the contents of a ' mirror world,' namely the part of the environment that is mirrored in consciousness. In accordance with this the evolutionary tendency seems to be to keep even this most elementary basis of reactions, the ' mirror ' or perceptual world, plastic and adaptable towards ever new demands, just as our ideas are adaptable and flexible. And according to the results of the theory of perceptions put forward here, which is based on the eidetic investigations, the two spheres are very closely connected.

Pedagogical experiment leads us along the same lines ;

for it has been shown in exhaustive statistical surveys (*vide* above) that the eidetic phase and the whole mental structure accompanying it, in particular the perceptual structure peculiar to it, are preserved longer than usual in children who are educated by methods adapted to the mentality of youth.[1]

The founders and protagonists of the modern *Arbeitsschule* held extremely optimistic views as to the plasticity of the youthful mind. In particular they held that the higher mental life is intimately bound up with the sensory sphere, and that it is therefore necessary to take account of this connection in all attempts at guiding the youthful mind. Here, then, they receive far-reaching justification for their views.[2]

The close coupling of perceptions and phenomena that are close to perceptions with the structures of the higher mental life, also provides us with an appropriate entrance gate for investigating the higher mental life of various types. For this purpose we use the combined methods of *experimental*

---

[1] This should explain why M. Zillig, during her investigations in Würzburg, found an exceptional number of eidetic subjects in *Hilfsschulen* (schools for mentally defectives). *Fortschritte der Psychologie*, edited by Karl Marbe, Vol. V, 1922. In the *Hilfsschule* the principle of the 'object-lesson' stands far more generally and more exclusively in the forefront. In normal schools it has not yet been introduced to anything like the same extent.

[2] This connection has been dissolved by the centuries long domination of rationalistic philosophies, chiefly under the influence of the doctrine of lower and higher psychic capacity, which is being more and more widely accepted. One of the results of this doctrine is the division of the Kantian critique of reason into transcendental æsthetics and transcendental logic. But fundamental philosophical conceptions have always had a profound repercussion on pedagogic views. As against this, there has always been a close connection between 'sensuality' and 'sense' in the mind of artists, who, even in this respect akin to the child's type of mind, have held themselves aloof from the influence of philosophical theories. How close this connection is must be clear to anyone who, for instance, tries to approach Goethe's inner world, through the medium of Gundolf's penetrating book.

C

and structural psychology, which are, as it were, a combination of the experimental method and the philosophic (*geisteswissenschaftliche*) procedure advocated chiefly by E. Spranger. It consists in bringing to the consciousness of our various types of subjects their peculiar modes of experience, by means of the perceptual phenomena and phenomena related to perception that can be produced experimentally. Without this, the subjects would not become aware of such experiences. In this way we can show them, as it were, various outer forts of their inner life, draw their attention to its characteristics and stimulate them to speak about it.[1]

The perceptions and the phenomena closely related to perceptions are not connected only with the superposed strata of the higher mental life, but also with their own deeper and even more elementary basis, the bodily organization. They are therefore the appropriate starting-point for investigations of the *psycho-physical personality*, and are a particularly delicate reagent.[2]

If a large number of young eidetic subjects is examined, two types clearly differentiate themselves among cases of approximately equal strength : those who have E.Is. that are close to A.Is. (*nachbildnahe*), and those whose E.Is. follow the laws of memory images more closely (*vorstellungsnahe*). (Once more it must be remembered that all E.Is. are literally *visible*.) The A.I.-like E.Is. have only a slender connection (' integration ') with the rest of the mental life, but like ordinary A.Is. they are dependent to a high degree on the

[1] For details see ' *Grundformen menschlichen Seins*,' Berlin, 1930. Naturally it is chiefly adults that are used for such observations.

[2] Cf. for the following remarks : Walther Jaensch, " Über psychophysische Konstitutionstypen." *Münchener Med. Wochenschr.* 1921, No. 35, and *Monatsschr. f. Kinderheilk.* Vol. 22, 1921. Also the monograph by Walther Jaensch, *Grundzüge einer Physiologie und Klinik der Psychophysischen Persönlichkeit*, Berlin, 1926.

physiological conditions of sensory stimulation. Just as in A.Is., their clearness depends above all on whether one point of the picture was fixated, and for how long. Furthermore, they are chiefly dependent on the intensity of the colours, the presence of extensive, homogeneously coloured parts in the picture, the sharpness of the contours and similar, *purely sensory* factors. On the other hand, they do not depend at all—or only to a very small extent—on the interest aroused by the picture. Even in cases of medium strength they are complementary to the original picture ; only in the strongest cases have they got the same colours. These E.Is. usually appear in two dimensions, even if the original test-object was three-dimensional. Only in exceptional cases do they stand out three-dimensionally in space. How completely these E.Is. are split off from the rest of the personality is evident from the fact that the subject can only with difficulty produce changes in the content of the E.Is. by a voluntary effort of the imagination, and in the extreme limiting case (which is rare, however), cannot influence them at all. Even where such changes can be carried out to any extent, they are bound in a striking manner to the colour material that has been given through fixation. In fact they can only be carried out more or less slowly and sometimes not without effort, by re-forming, transposing, or 'rekneading' the colour material. Their thorough-going dissociation from the total personality (or small ' integration ' with it) is also evident from the fact that in pronounced cases that have easily produced, numerous, and intense E.Is. of this type, they are felt as foreign bodies in the mental life, as something alien to the personality and sometimes as positive hindrances. We had a boy under observation, who could only learn lessons by heart early in the morning, because he otherwise relived everything he had seen during the day in the form of small pictures of this rigid type between the lines, and was unable to get rid of them. Moreover, he did not belong to those cases that are constitutionally determined and therefore pathological in the true sense of the word. He has developed very well both bodily and mentally.

The existence of these rigid E.Is. does not depend on their respective contents being thought about. They can therefore not be removed by giving another direction to thinking and the flow of ideas. Their disappearance rather gives the impression of a purely *optical*-physiological process, as in the case of A.Is. In the weaker cases, or in those of medium strength, it is clear that they vanish in much the same way as A.Is. Their colour content begins to vanish, now here, now there, often in separate ' clouds.'

If eidetic subjects are examined in large numbers, one soon comes across cases in which one enters a different world, as it were. The opposite to what has been discussed above is true of them. Moreover, *pure* cases of this type seem to be more frequent than *pure* cases of the previous type. The E.Is. are now no longer regarded as foreign, something that forces itself upon the personality from the outside, but as something belonging to the self ; not as an annoyance, which one would like to throw off, but as a *gift*, often as an intimate, loved possession that one wants to retain. While the E.Is. that were described above are, like A.Is., dissociated from the mental personality, these E.Is., like the contents of the imaginal life, are closely bound up with it, with this *one* exception, that they, too, are always literally visible to the eyes. Like memory images, their colours always correspond to those of the real objects or test pictures. They never appear in complementary colours, and if the test-object was three-dimensional, the E.Is., too, are three-dimensional. They are as flexible and changeable as memory images, willingly and smoothly following every change in the flow of ideas. Their occurrence, stability and disappearance hardly depend on sense-physiological or optical factors at all, but most decisively on psychological factors. Fixation of the test picture is unnecessary and even a hindrance. On the contrary, the picture or object should be inspected with an unforced, sweeping glance, which makes the attentive perception of all the details possible. If the colouring is homogeneous, or at any rate similar in large parts of the picture, it presents favourable conditions for the first type of E.Is., but not for the second. For these, the best picture is one rich in detail, which keeps attention and interest alive. The quality and completeness of the E.Is. is within wide limits independent of the time of inspection, but depends far more on whether the test picture has some reference to the interests of the observer, because ' selection ' and choice from the point of view of fixed interests takes place in these eidetic phenomena just as in the mental sphere. The E.I. vanishes and reappears according as the observer directs his attention to or away from the contents portrayed in the E.I. Like memory images, and unlike the E.Is. first described, these E.Is. appear and vanish as a whole. Changes can be made in the image that have no basis in the colour of the original, and cannot be achieved by any ' re-kneading ' of the colours. They take place as promptly as the change of ideas, and without the effort of a ' re-kneading process.' Corresponding to the free and rapid changes in imaginal contents, all sorts of transformations usually take place spontaneously within these E.Is., particularly if they persist somewhat longer than usual. To start with, these changes are closely based

on the original. Again, just as is the case in changes in the
imaginal contents, they always have *meaning* in some way,
e.g. they will continue the events or actions portrayed in the
original. Even where they remodel these in some phantastic
way, they nevertheless always start from the inner relations
of that which has been portrayed and not from the colour
material. These relations are then remodelled and taken over
into the new picture. In a word, they never lack intelligible
' meaning.' The transformations that take place in E.Is.
of the first type consist of changes in the form of ' spatial
transposition,' doubling, overlaying and similar processes
that lack ' meaning.'

Where these two totally different types of image occur,
we are also dealing with totally different types of mind. The
mental organism of individuals with A.I.-like E.Is. is in
extreme cases fitted together out of pieces, as it were, like a
machine ; the individuals with labile E.Is., which stand
closer to memory images, in pronounced cases present an
organic unity in which the component parts are from the
start in closest connection and interaction. In this type the
mental functions interpenetrate, as it were ; in the other
they behave as though dissociated from one another. *E.g.*
corresponding to the E.Is. that force themselves on the
observer's notice, and persist even against his will, there can
be ideas that seem no less alien to the personality and are
felt as foreign bodies like the E.Is.

As regards somatic characteristics, too, there is a distinct
difference between these pure types. In the first type, the
A.I.-like E.Is. point to a heightened sensitivity of the optic
sensorial nerves and their nearest connections in the central
organ. Entirely corresponding to this we find an increase
in the sensitivity of motor nerves to electrical and mechanical

stimulation (the so-called Erbs phenomenon, *facialis* phenomenon of various degrees, etc.) as well as a lowering of the
different sensory and sensible thresholds to the same stimuli,
as compared with the corresponding conditions beyond the
eidetic phase of development and in adults. The eyes are
chiefly characterized by their contrast to those of the other
type, which has a large, lustrous eye. But in this type it is
particularly noticeable that all those characteristics of youth
are missing, which have been expressed in the phrase ' the
large eyes of a child.' Their eyes are small, deep-set, comparatively lifeless, without lustre, with no ' soulful ' expression. The eyes thus also seem to betray that dissociation
of functions and organic systems within the mental sphere,
just as the motor expressions, which often remind one of an
automaton or a machine. In very pronounced cases there
may also be present a peculiar, ' pinched ' facial expression,
which probably also rests on hypersensitivity and which, in
its extreme form, is known to medical men as the ' tetany
face.'

It is clear, not only from this symptom, but also from the
above-mentioned increase in sensitivity, that we are dealing
with a normal youthful type, whose pathologic form is the
tetanoid condition, for this is predominantly characterized by
changes in sensitivity as described above. Moreover, the
characteristics of this type of personality, including the
eidetic phenomena peculiar to it, are susceptible to feeding
with calcium, a treatment that is also recommended for
tetany (*hypothyreosis*). Their E.Is. can be diminished or
extinguished by calcium feeding. This result is particularly
impressive when in pronounced cases of this kind all phenomena, including A.Is., at first only occur in original colours,
and then, under the influence of calcium, which suppresses

or diminishes their basic disposition, take on complementary colours, so that *e.g.* negative A.Is., *i.e.* A.Is. in complementary colours, occur for the first time, after having been incapable of excitation before. But we must always remember that, with the exception of over-pronounced cases, we are here only characterizing a definite youthful phase of development, that is, a *normal* youthful type, whose characteristics usually diminish in strength later on, as does the supernormal sensitivity.

A further proof that we are dealing here with normal manifestations of youth and not with pathological cases, is to be found in the fact that the other type is similarly related to symptoms known to medical practice, only in a different way ; and this in spite of the fact that its lower stages embody all that we are wont to regard and to hold in esteem as expressing true, carefree youth. One of the characteristics of this type are the large eyes.[1] According to the particular personality, they may be lustrous or dreamily veiled ; but we can find a continuous transition into those protuberant eyes known as ' *protrusio bulbi*,' which are one of the most striking symptoms of *Basedow's disease*.[2] The lively play of the pupils and the ' soulful ' expression, reflect the personality to the outside world, as it were ; we feel that it presents us with a true mirror of the continually fluctuating inner world of youth. At the same time, however, these scintillating eyes are the partial expression of a heightened sensibility of the vegetative nervous system, and in particular of its quickened response to mental stimuli. Both of these are symptoms that are similar to those met with in basedowoid

[1] Compare, *e.g.* the two screen-types, " Micky " and " Jackie Coogan." [Trans.]

[2] Better known in England as *Graves' disease*.

conditions, where they are more pronounced still. Apart from the moist, luminous eye, there is a large number of other symptoms pointing to heightened vegetative sensitivity, particularly to mental stimuli. Vasomotor processes and the pulse are easily affected, especially by mental, but also by bodily conditions ; arythmic respiration, that is, changes in the frequency of the pulse during breathing, strong tendency to perspire, etc., are common. Individuals of this type are predominantly gracefully built, and have a soft, satin or silky skin with a low resistance to electric currents. The thyroid gland is often slightly enlarged. All these symptoms, or rather their exaggeration, belong to the basedowoid condition. This complex of characteristics, with its attendant eidetic phenomena, cannot be influenced by calcium, even during prolonged treatment.

To indicate the relation of these two types to well-known clinical conditions (Tetany, neuropathic Basedow), we call the first, ' T-type,' the second, ' B-type.' This corresponds to the constitution already observed in the clinic for inner medicine of G. v. Bergmann from an aetiological standpoint, and called by him " stigmatization in the vegetative nervous system." But this constitutional type attains a new and far more general significance from these psycho-physiological investigations. For it must be remembered that these symptoms, within the limits attained in our subjects, *are merely normal physiological characteristics of a certain youthful stage of development*, and in no way pathological manifestations.

Really pure types, with which we had to start our investigations and the above descriptions, are comparatively rare. The great majority of cases is an ' amalgam ' of the B and the T characteristics. But on the basis of the knowledge obtained through a study of the rare *pure* types, it is possible to separate the characteristics appertaining to these two types quite clearly in each individual case of the mixed types. The proportion of each type of characteristic present can be determined in part by rigorously quantitative tests. This will already indicate why the group of workers here place so much emphasis on the investigation of *pure* types, although these are comparatively rare.[1]

If some psychologists and medical men occasionally still look askance at the results obtained from such single instances, it shows up once more the one-sided orientation of the younger biological sciences towards the older inorganic sciences. Physics and chemistry do not take individual cases into account, certain related sciences, like geophysics, solar physics, etc., excepted. Here, in every investigation that is to have a more general significance, any object of investigation, *e.g.* a substance that is to be chemically analysed, must be replaceable by an unlimited number of substances of the same kind. But Ewald Hering had already been tireless in affirming that few things had retarded the progress of biological science as much as the one-sided application to it of the habits of thought developed by the inorganic sciences.[2] It is quite compatible with this assertion, of course, that the biological sciences will always have to be grateful to be able to make extensive loans from their physical and chemical neighbours, wherever such loans are in place. Indeed, in some fields they will themselves remain physical or chemical science. Ewald Hering and his school also emphasized that the pro-

[1] At any rate that is true of the conditions here. But the distribution of types varies according to locality and race. We must therefore expect that conditions are different elsewhere. Indeed, according to some recent investigations, it seems extremely probable that the pure B-type is sometimes far more numerous.

[2] Cf. *e.g.* F. B. Hoffmann, " Ewald Hering," *Münchener med. Wochenschrift*, 1918, also M. Verworn, *Allgemeine Physiologie*, 5th edition, 1909.

perties of living processes differing from those of the inorganic processes in nature, are most clearly manifested in the highest levels, the psychophysiological processes. That is why such an important place was given to the physiology of the senses in general physiology.[1] For the same reason the individual differentiation of living processes can be most clearly seen in psychophysiology,[2] although differentiation is a very much

[1] Cf. *e.g.* A. v. Tschermak, *Allgemeine Physiologie*, I, 1924.

[2] It is still usual in our subject to speak of the teachings about the relationships between mind and body as ' psychophysics.' But the time has come to substitute for this word, which has actually become misleading, the word ' psychophysiology.' This means immeasurably more than a mere terminological distinction : it means the plan and the roadnet of future research. The term ' psychophysics ' was appropriate in the older stage of our science, when it had to seek support from physics for its teachings about the relations between mind and body, because the as yet undeveloped biological sciences could not give any assistance. To-day, ' psychophysics ' is a catchword, which, in the eyes of outsiders, merely serves the purpose of giving the stamp of an ostensibly recognized science to certain dilettantisms, that are almost unspoilt by biological or psychological thinking and knowledge, as long as they appear outwardly in the guise of physics. Our science will progress in the near future by going hand in hand with the sciences of life (in the widest sense), which are her nearest neighbours. The investigations that are merely reported in a very short and dogmatic form here are intended as contributions to this programme. The friendly and neighbourly relations with physics will not be severed by this scheme, just as little as they were between physiology and physics when the former, particularly since E. Hering's time, remembered that it had a right of its own and ceased wanting to be merely applied physics and chemistry. This procedure should gradually banish the prejudice and antipathy against psychology, which is widespread in certain circles. It should also dispose of the idea that psychology is inimical to philosophy. For all these prejudices are the result of an idea, derived from the older psychophysics, that psychology falsifies our picture of mental life by simply taking over the methods of thought developed in the inorganic sciences. Those who were interested in drawing a pure picture made philosophy their ally, for it has no part in this carrying over of concepts, or falsification, as it was called. It was largely the fault of this psychological ' physicism ' that to many philosophers ' scientific ' (in the sense of ' natural science ') has come to be synonymous with ' construing,' ' far removed from reality.' This view is even hinted at in Rickert's " *Über die Grenzen der natur- wissenschaftlichen Begriffsbildung,*" a significant work in many respects. Rickert here represents the concepts of natural science as a system of thought striving to recede and far removed from reality.

more widely distributed property of life. Progress is only possible in this field if we take ' types ' into consideration ; and if we wish to investigate types, we must start from the pure cases. The mass of individual cases can then be understood as compounded of these pure cases in varying proportions. That is the reason why *geisteswissenschaftliche* (philosophical) psychology, which never allowed itself to be led astray by the example of inorganic science, has practised this method as though it were a commonplace hardly in need of discussion, cf. the " *Lebensformen* " of E. Spranger, who continues the tradition of the Dilthey school in this book.

To Dilthey the final goal of historical studies was always the penetration of the *highest levels* of the mind of man. Their individual aspects are not expressed in *pure* forms in any arbitrary number of individuals that could be selected at random, just as we might select subjects for experiments on thresholds from any lecture-room : they appear only once or twice in the course of centuries. Nevertheless, the description and interpretation of Goethe, for instance, in the only sense that is justifiable in the highest mental levels, has a *general* significance—although anyone prosecuting research on Goethe would be completely at a loss if he were to be asked how many ' cases of Goethe ' he had found. The general significance lies in the fact that Goethe has already experienced, in a purer and clearer form, what all or most of us feel in a confused way under the same circumstances in life. That is why many of us often take up Goethe again, or, since most of us belong to a ' mixed type,' we take up some other ' *pure* feeling type,' *e.g.* George or Eichendorff. However, let us leave these high regions and return to the fruitful valleys ! Here we shall no longer find the rare alpine species in isolated specimens ; but, instead we shall find a rich selection of field flowers. Although we are dealing with average lives here, we shall be able to collect a far greater number that conforms to the pure types than the investigator of the highest levels, where there is a far greater individual differentiation. Nevertheless, even in our region the number of *pure* types is small in relation to the great mass of cases ; but their importance lies in their enabling us to analyse this mass, and to understand it as an amalgamation of the pure types. We can look upon it as a B-T group, in which sometimes the B component, at other times the T component predominates. Calcium therapy has shown that this is actually the case. As this treatment only affects the T complex, it is very often possible to suppress the T characteristics, including the E.Is. peculiar to them, so that only the B complex and its characteristic E.Is. remain. In this way it can be proved that the original condition was a combination of both B and T characteristics.

Some investigators have found it strange that we have not made more of this division into types in our experimental work on the normal structure of perceptions and images. In the interests of researches that had been planned, we have been asked which type is to be preferred for that kind of work. The answer is contained in what has been said above. In the majority of youthful eidetic subjects, *both* components are present. We must therefore regard the state in which they are so coupled together as the normal state in youth, and use it as the basis on which investigations of the structure of perceptions and images are carried out. If, in investigations of this kind, all the more pronounced cases are grouped together without distinction, one will only rarely find cases that deviate markedly from the majority because of the purity of their type. In practice only the pure B-type is found to be relatively frequent, and, as we mentioned at the beginning of our monograph on the structure of perceptions, cases of this type were, in fact, at first excluded from our investigations, because they differed from the majority of cases in several respects. As we have mentioned in the work just cited, and have indicated above, observations have been made suggesting that the pure B-type may be much more frequent under conditions differing widely from those prevalent here, particularly among different races.

The pure T-type is much rarer. Moreover, in the strongly pronounced cases, which are always particularly instructive, there is usually some admixture of the other component. This is specially true of children, among whom the absolutely pure types are much rarer than among adults—which again shows that the normal characteristic of youth is the interlocking of both types. All this, again, justifies the symbolic representation we gave of eidetic images. The E.Is. of the pure T-type resemble A.Is., those of the pure B-type M.Is. But they are also optical phenomena, and literally *visible*. The E.Is. of youthful eidetic subjects, therefore, lie in general on a line connecting these end-points, as we have pointed out before.[1] This property of E.Is. again expresses the fact that the B-T complex is the normal type in youth.

In the interests of scientific and practical progress, we must keep questions of type and constitution clear of considerations of value ; they must be treated purely scientifically, *i.e.* psychologically and psychophysiologically. ' Disease ' is not

---

[1] Our contention that there is an inner connection between E.Is., A.Is., and M.Is., has been questioned (cf. Allport, *Brit. Journ. Psych.*, 1924), but in answer we would point out the empirically proven fact, that E.Is. in general occupy an intermediate position between A.Is. and M.Is., having properties that sometimes approximate to the one and sometimes to the other.

a purely scientific term ; it always includes the concept of value. Whenever the term ' disease ' is connected with ' type ' or ' constitution,' it only refers to one-sided, disharmonic and imperfectly balanced forms of the type. Such individuals fall below the normal requirements of life in some respect or other. To discuss the problem of types merely from the negative point of view of value or non-value is quite one-sided, for it is just as important to bring it into relation with the positively valuable aspect of natural science. It is this aspect which is of particular interest to the teacher. He wants to know what typical characteristics of personality can call forth greater achievements, and what characteristics are developed best by methods of education adapted to the needs of the child. We have mentioned above that this kind of education keeps the eidetic characteristics of youth alive for a much longer time. We can now add that above all it favours the lively, mobile B-type characteristics, which are found to be widely prevalent under such conditions, and must therefore be encouraged by them. This is quite understandable, since the eidetic world of this type stands close to M.Is. and manifests a rich imagination. These observations, however, only apply to the school period, chiefly to the years up to the end of the primary school. We must allow the possibility that in later life a stronger measure of T characteristics in addition to the others may be valuable, since they give to the mind a greater rigidity and, perhaps, ' backbone ' ; to the ambitious they give a more clearly defined direction.

Those who believed the eidetic researches to be no more than an analysis of E.Is., are very far removed indeed from an understanding of the purpose of these investigations. If that were the case, then it would indeed be a very profound narrowing of our mental horizon to expect that a field, whose investigation was more or less started by chance, could provide a basis for so many other psychological researches. But E.Is. are, in truth, merely the most obvious sign of the structure of personality normal to youth. They are the most easily accessible outer fortress for our penetration into a phase of development that has hitherto hardly been noticed, in which the building up of our world of perceptions and ideas takes place and which, therefore, at a later period gives to what we call ' our world ' its formal stamp. The peculiar perceptual world of the eidetic phase, and particularly the type of thinking and feeling that accompanies it, have not been taken into account either by theory or by pedagogic practice—except for the tactful intuition of a few pedagogues. These questions, however, go far beyond the fundamental discussions from the point of view of educational practice that ought to be given ; they must therefore be reserved for a later publication. In this work there is only room for indicating a few of the conclusions that have been reached in some of the investigations, which, we believe, are of great importance to education.

The whole of these investigations throws new light on the question of the so-called ' pedagogic intellectualism,' round which discussion at present centres. There can be no doubt that there are profound reasons for the reform of the universities at present being carried out by the Secretary of State, Herr Becker, as well as the reorganization of the system of higher education by the Minister of Education, Herr Boelitz and his officials. Both are aimed against that ' intellectualism,' of which the older systems have so often been accused. But the justification for this criticism can only be found by means of penetrating researches into the psychology of childhood. We are far from expecting immediate practical results from such researches, although several results have been obtained already, which encourage further work along these lines. But the less foreseen such facts are, and the further they digress from accepted views, the more important becomes our duty of first perfecting them within the body of psychology, before asking practical men to try them out. All who are at work on the new psychology of childhood should keep before them the maxims of the great Descartes : in pure research one should not recoil from radical doubt and re-orientation ; but we should be more careful where the institutions of Life are concerned, which, like heavy bodies, are difficult to raise up when they are lying on the ground, and are even difficult to hold up when they begin to totter.

The doctrines and institutions of educational practice have always been dependent on current philosophies. This is true whether the men engaged in educational practice have sought counsel from philosophy herself, or whether their basic philosophic views and attitude have come to them along the countless and often untraceable channels of general culture, which is, as we know, always founded on some ' *Weltanschauung*.' Now if we take a bird's-eye view of the systems prevalent during the last centuries—leaving out of account a few smaller and less important counter-currents— we see that *rationalistic* systems of thought entirely predominate. The great philosophic systems, in which the conception of life that underlies the prevailing culture is always mirrored most faithfully, to a great extent see in some form of logic the deepest and finally directive discipline. This conception appears in two substantially different forms. In the one, the thought process as conceived by the science of logic is regarded as giving to our whole method of acquiring knowledge, and, therefore, to our whole specifically human conception of the world, its deepest basis and final justification. At the same time it lays down the forms that reality has to assume in order to become an object for knowledge (logic as a system of 'innate ideas' or 'rational truths,' or even as 'transcendental logic').

But the basic rationalistic hypothesis also appears in a second and more far-reaching form. Thought as conceived by the science of logic is not only regarded as laying down the forms and foundations for our methods of acquiring knowledge, and therefore for our conception of the world : Being, and the world, are themselves regarded as the products of such thought ('metaphysical logic' and 'logical Idealism'). The systems of Descartes, Spinoza, Leibniz, Kant, Hegel, and the Neo-Kantians conform to one or other of these types, or to both. There have been a few opposite tendencies ; but they have had no deeper influence. Such are some elements of Leibnizian philosophy diverging from rationalism, which have up to quite recently been almost unnoticed ; the fundamental conceptions of Schelling, which, though they are false in some respects, are nevertheless of the greatest importance ; even Kant in the *Critique of Judgment* and Kant as a metaphysical thinker, whom only the most recent historical research is again beginning to bring to light (Max Wundt,[1] H. Heimsoeth).

Since the basis of pedagogy is determined by current

---

[1] Max Wundt, " *Kant als Metaphysiker*," Stuttgart, 1924. Peter Petersen pointed out to me that Rousseau in particular seems to have belonged to that extreme eidetic type, which we have been investigating, and that this decisively influenced his philosophy as well as his educational system. Petersen is attempting to show that the same is true of Wilhelm Wundt, in the excellent work on this investigator and thinker, which has just appeared. (*Frommans Klassiker der Philosophie :* P. Petersen, " *W. Wundt und seine Zeit*," Stuttgart, 1925.)

philosophies, educational practice necessarily took logic as its model. Since the beginnings of logic in Aristotle, it has been bound up with grammar. Hence in the schools the ideal of the logician was often fused with that of the grammarian. This is not altered by the fact that logic was only rarely taught in the school. The point is that it expressed a *tendency*, and it is that that we are here seeking to express in an extreme form. Where this tendency predominates, the subjects that are taught appear as a framework of logic filled in with facts. Inner participation is not directed to the subject, but to the form of thought (formula, rule), which it expresses. Let us hasten to add that in criticizing this ideal of the logician we are not criticizing the logical thinker, nor do we criticize grammar in this ideal of the grammarian.[1] The pedagogical ideal of the logician rests on the untrue assumption that productive logical thinking proceeds *because* of the laws of logic and also has its psychological basis in them, since it proceeds *in accordance* with them and its *results* agree with them. The investigations into the structure of personality of the child in the eidetic phase of development have shown—if we may be allowed to summarize the pedagogically most important result in a few words—that the closest parallel to the structure of personality of the child is not the mental structure of the logician, but that of the artist.[2] If we advocate that these facts should be recognized, we by no means wish to advocate or to start a culture of æstheticism, or a weakening of logical thinking. Productive

[1] Nor do we wish to say anything against Logic as a science. But Logic cannot teach us to think. This has already been strongly emphasized by one logician, Wilhelm Schuppe, in his acute works on Logic and Epistemology, which do not deserve to be forgotten.

[2] For more details see our monograph (in preparation), " *Über das Wesen der Kunst und die Kunst des Kindes*," Benno Filser, Augsburg.

logical thinking, even in the most exact sciences, is far more closely related to the type of mind of the artist and the child than the ideal of the logician would lead us to suppose. That is shown in the loving attention to the matter in hand, in that close union of object and subject in children and artists, of which eidetic phenomena are merely a particularly evident expression. It is shown in the fusion of the person with the object, so that every lifeless system of signs ranged in between is felt to be a hindrance. The grammatical structures of language are such a system of signs, unless concrete imagination infuses life into them. Only psychological research can discover how the thinking process takes place. Logic represents to us thoughts arranged in their inner order and deduces one from the other; but if we examine the autobiographies of successful scientists, we find that productive thinking must have a close relation to artistic production. Read, for instance, H. Poincaré's own description of his work, or Hilbert's enthusiastic description of the irresistible attraction of mathematical research, or the thoughts put forward at the opening of the congress for internal specialists in Vienna by Wenckebach,[1] who is a strong adherent of the strictest school of experimental physiology. He believed most firmly that it was in the interests of the progress of his science that educational methods, even in the natural sciences and in medicine, should again begin to take their departure from the mentality of the artist and the child.

The ' intellectualism ' of the older school system does not lie so much in the emphasis laid on certain subjects (*e.g.* the sciences in the university), as in the predominance of the

---

[1] F. Wenckebach, speech read at the opening of the 35th congress for inner medicine in Vienna, 1923. *Verhandlungen d. deutschen Gesellschaft f. innere Medizin*, published by A. Géronne, Munich, 1923; cf. also our essay, " Zum Gedächtnis von Alois Riehl," *Kantstudien*, 1923.

logician's ideal, which permeates all the subjects equally. A really fundamental change in this respect is not to be expected so much from new curricula or a readjustment of the relative importance of different subjects in the universities, as from the substitution for that misleading ideal of more correct conceptions about the psychology of thinking, particularly the thinking of the child. It will certainly always stand to the credit of our leading officials that they correctly pointed out a weak aspect of the older educational system. But the over-emphasis of some subjects and the comparative neglect of others was only one of its minor faults. The reform of education, which will have to come about sooner or later, will have to be far more fundamental and will need a far profounder psychological basis. This basis has still to be built by science.[1] The natural sciences, even mathematics

---

[1] It is for this reason that we in nowise intend any criticism by the above discussion. Many excrescences of the "*Jugendbewegung*" (league of youth)—which in itself is a very admirable movement—are due to the fact that the lack of clearness as to the precise meaning of the concept 'intellectualism,' to which we have alluded, is particularly widespread there, and has had some very unfortunate practical consequences. Youth, however, is increasingly overcoming this uncertainty and at the same time achieving a firmer and clearer realization of its work in life. Some years ago, there used to be much talk in one of the organs of such a group of seekers after new paths, from whom the author expects much, about 'forbidden vocations,' particularly with reference to the 'intellectualism' that had to be fought, but also for other reasons. I am very pleased to see many of the vocations that formerly were either 'forbidden,' or at any rate looked upon with disfavour, being warmly advocated in the pages of that same organ by young people who have taken up some of these vocations and are trying to infuse into them the spirit of their movement. They are beginning to realize that the 'intellectualism' and the lack of nobility did not lie in the vocations themselves, but in the way in which they were carried on. The case of school subjects is probably very similar. When I was writing these lines, I heard a very experienced teacher (Dr Hölk, director of the *Gymnasium* in Marburg) say in a lecture that he had had many pupils belonging to various groups of the *Jugendbewegung* and had seen that even they could derive pleasure from the so-called rational subjects, even from grammar. But everything had to be concrete (*anschaulich*), not dead and

and grammar, can be treated without 'intellectualism';
poetry and the arts can be treated 'intellectualistically.'
This may not be taken to mean that the solution is to be
found in an 'innate ability to teach.' There will always be
differences in the ability of teachers; that is so obvious as
hardly to need mentioning. The important point is that the
average standard must be raised. To-day even a bad writer
probably writes better than many a noted author before the
time of Goethe. There can be no doubt that a lot of changes
will take place in education when incorrect conceptions about
the processes of thought are replaced by more correct ones.
Moreover, it cannot be objected that this would not reach
to the root of the matter, because teachers have never been
much concerned with psychology or philosophy, whether of
the right or wrong kind. All teaching is based on psychological cenceptions. Unless a personality with pronounced
youthful characteristics, in other words a 'born teacher,'
instinctively strikes out newer and better paths, the conceptions of an almost superseded rationalistic philosophy will
be the guiding ones, and these conceptions are infused into
us from the total culture around us. As the psychiatrist

abstract. That is the whole crux of the matter! Almost any subject can
be purified of this 'intellectualism,' which is such a bugbear. In this
connection we might mention the efforts of M. Deutschbein to relate the
grammar of foreign languages to the forms of thinking and the type of
thinker of a foreign people, and to introduce this point of view, which
surely is close to life, into his English grammar for schools. If we have
been informed correctly, it seems that even in our sphere of work we have
been accused of 'intellectualism.' The greater emphasis that is being
laid on psychology in philosophy is even said to be partly responsible for
this 'intellectualism.' It cannot be denied that the way in which psychological work was carried out during a short phase of its development, lends
some support to these accusations. But that was not the fault of psychology. In the whole field of science there is to-day probably no subject
which is more full of vitality, and probably nothing that is farther removed
from the one-sidedness of intellectualism and more strongly concerned in
working against it.

R. Sommer has pointed out, these conceptions not only dominate the theory of teaching, but also our codes of law and therefore the administration of law.

Pedagogy, more than any other science, is interested in discovering and taking into consideration those factors of thinking that are part of the mentality of the artist and that have been overlooked by rationalistic psychology. The eidetic investigations have already shown that the closest resemblance to the mind of the child is not the mental structure of the logician, but that of the artist. In fact there are to be found among artists numerous personalities that permanently keep the characteristics of the youthful eidetic phase of development. For this reason it is advisable for educational purposes that the characteristics of youthful, eidetic personalities, which are at the same time characteristics of many artists, should be observed and taken into account.[1] The extraordinary successes of the painter Erwin Heckmann in the *deutsches Landerziehungsheim* (German educational institute in the country) in Castle Ettersburg, are due to his using and preserving the mental characteristics of the eidetic phase in the children. When these characteristics, which are so prevalent in childhood, are used and kept alive, one finds an extraordinarily high percentage, in fact the majority of children, achieving results in drawing, painting and the plastic arts that are acknowledged to have artistic value by all who have seen them. The same is true, as R. Nolte found to our surprise in the Marburg North school, of the invention of fairy tales.[2] In a different, yet somewhat

[1] The monograph of O. Kroh, "*Subjektive Anschauungsbilder bei Jugendlichen*" (Göttingen, 1922), contains valuable suggestions from an educational point of view, based on the first investigations of the eidetic phase of development.

[2] "*Analyse der freien Märchenproduktion bei Schulkindern*," Dr. Phil. dissertation, Marburg, 1925.

similar way my former assistant A. Kobusch has utilized these faculties in the lower and even in the middle classes of the *Gymnasium Paulinum* in Münster. If the results obtained were limited to education in art, these attempts could only be of importance as an experiment so far as education in general is concerned, which does not consist in raising a generation of artists or founding a purely æsthetic culture. But the results go far beyond that, provided the conditions of co-operation with other subjects are fulfilled, or at any rate, provided the other subjects do not exercise any retarding opposition. Once the creative powers are freed in one direction, which, in this particular case, has been shown by our investigations to be wholly peculiar to the world of youth ; once the shackles of school passivity are broken at one point, a kind of inner liberation, the awakening of a higher activity, generally sets in.[1] Above all, to the eidetic phase of development, as well as to the mentality of the artist, there belongs a peculiar structure of the mental powers, particularly of thinking ; and the arousing and vivifying of these powers benefit all the subjects taught, even the most rigorously logical.

These investigations, however, also have purely theoretical applications. They give us important starting-points for investigating and solving a number of problems that are very much discussed to-day.

The Berlin group of ' *Gestalt* ' psychologists are very

---

[1] There are great parallels to this small, but significant process. Gundolf, with delicate intuition, has shown how Herder was the first to encourage the youthful Goethe in freely developing the creative powers that had long been lying dormant, and to dare to express the neologisms, which differed so much from traditional practice. It was Herder who freed Goethe from the shackles of ' cultural passivity,' as we might call the attitude towards environment and its cultural contents, in analogy to ' school passivity.'

emphatic in their advocacy of a doctrine, which, they claim, has revolutionized psychology and made obsolete a great deal of previous work, so that it is really the beginning of all scientific, psychological and philosophic work.[1] Such far-reaching claims are probably unique in the history of science, and they must therefore expect to be rigorously tested and then answered without reserve. The main body of this theory was at first made up of speculations about the physics of cerebral processes, which were supposed to underlie the perception of *Gestalt*. Latterly, its supporters have placed less emphasis on these hypotheses, but more on the quite general assertion that not elements or disjunct pieces, but ' *Gestalten*,' are the primary basis of mental life, and by ' *Gestalten* ' they understood wholes and relations. Therefore not even sensations and perceptions are primary, as sensationism used to think, but the relations in which they occur.

But in its generalized form this doctrine is neither true nor new. It is not new : for the whole tradition from Plato and Aristotle to psychovitalism, and the whole of philosophic idealism, had looked upon *relations* as more primary than elements; moreover, in scientific psychology in the narrower sense, relations have long ago received a wide recognition that goes beyond generalities and has proved its fruitfulness in scientific research. Now these efforts were cautious, and they kept strictly to facts; moreover, the theory of elements has long been discarded. If, then, the Berlin ' *Gestalt* ' theory is held to be so important because of its simple and radical inversion of the element hypothesis, it must fail precisely because of its unsubtle, simple radicalism, as so many

---

[1] One occasionally even hears people, particularly in Berlin, speaking of " an era of *Gestalt* psychology."

of its forerunners have. Simple and oft repeated catchwords
will always spread in a sphere that interests many who are
not immediately connected with it, but is thoroughly known
only to few ; they are therefore the most effective, but at the
same time remain furthest from the real subtlety of things.
The facts are not so simple that one merely needs to invert
the thesis of sensationism, and to substitute relations for
' elements ' (sensations) as the more primary. The facts
protest against such a simple and easy procedure.

The methods for investigating types open up empirical
ways of approach to these problems, which have not been
recently discovered, but are as old as thought. The short
summary we have given above indicates that the closeness
with which elementary psychic processes depend on structures
of a higher order and on relations is variable. This interdependence is closer in the B-type than in the T-type. The
former, therefore, has the distinctive characteristics of the
organic to a higher degree than the latter, whose functions
are more mechanical. The dependence of sensory elements
on higher structures and on the total personality is above
all different at different levels of development. In the eidetic
phase of the child this interdependence is far closer than it is
in the case of adults. At this stage of development the sensations and perceptions are far more variable and ' plastic,'
according to the context in which they occur. They therefore
exhibit, in the most pronounced form, those phenomena which
have always been the cause for emphasizing relations and
wholes as opposed to elements, and for the assertion that
these ' wholes ' have a decisive influence on the so-called
psychic ' elements.' The facts that supported these theories
had hitherto been found purely from experiments on adults.
But now it is found that this influence of wholes on elements

is only present in a rudimentary form in adults, as compared with children and young people. We must therefore hope to find a solution for these ancient problems through child psychology.

Just as the dependence of elements on relations is not the same for different individuals and different stages of development, so it is not the same in all sense organs. During the eidetic phase of development this dependence is so close in the case of the eye, that the investigations of the structure of space perception actually furnish the empirical justification and explanation of certain central ideas of Kantian criticism, that is, of a doctrine whose chief content is this very assumption that the elements are decisively formed by structures of a higher order (*Anschauungsformen* and *Denkformen* in Kant himself, *Systemzusammenhänge* in neo-Kantianism).

In the ear, however, conditions are quite different. Here the facts all point to a far greater independence of sensory elements from wholes of higher order. It would therefore be merely obscuring the differences that exist here and the scientific problems arising out of them to assert that there are no exceptions to the dependence of elements on relations, just as sensationism formerly asserted that relations were without exception dependent on elements. This obscuring of scientific problems by some programmatic fundamental assumption is theoretically justified and fixed, as it were, by the physiological hypothesis of the *Gestalt* psychologists, which states that the relation of elements and relations is already laid down in the physical processes that seem to occur in all nervous and cerebral events, and may take place in all of them, as well as in inorganic nature, in the same way. But the relation of elements and relations within the various levels of reality, from the physical to the mental, is

by no means of the same kind, as it should be if this view
were correct. On the contrary, we find quite different forms
of this relation at various levels of reality and even at various
levels of the mind. It was the impression of a spiritual
reality, which had always led the older philosophies to oppose
a different conception of that relation to the one formed by
the inorganic sciences. If we wish to advance beyond those
philosophic formulations to a clearer knowledge of these facts,
we shall obtain the deepest insight into them in the psychological and its neighbouring, the psychophysiological spheres,
since the most widely different forms of the relation of elements to relations are to be found at their various levels.
Unless we want to ignore the most important contribution
that psychology and psychophysiology can make to these
questions, which are of such importance to our conceptions
of the world, we must start from exact empirical analysis of
the various forms of this relation at different levels of the
mental and in various functional types.

It seems to be this same typological method to which the
present advance of psychology along several lines is due ;
and it seems to be opening up strictly empirical methods of
approach to many problems. Among other achievements,
credit is also due to the physiologist, J. v. Kries, for having
emphasized, at a time when such advice was generally dis-
regarded, the great importance of insight into the logical and
methodological aspect for any real advance in science. One
of the great tasks of our time is to lay the foundations of the
sciences of organic nature, particularly in those branches in
which physical and chemical methods alone do not suffice,
however much we may continue to make grateful use of
them. The great times in which the sciences of inorganic
nature were established can be an example to us in our

attempts at solving the new problems, in so far as they teach us that such great advances can only be made if insight is gained simultaneously from the point of view of empirical science and from that of methodology. It is true that the literature of logic and epistemology gives us a certain initial support when, in the face of these new problems of the sciences of life, we hesitatingly have to follow paths that may lead us into conflict with our conscience, which has been trained in the school of the inorganic sciences.

The peculiar greatness of the times in which both mathematics and modern philosophy were born is due to the effective realization of that essential co-operation and intermingling of empirical and epistemological insight, which was to some extent lacking in the last epoch of the natural sciences. Instead of co-operation, we find to-day that the tendencies of science and epistemology are opposed. Hence the results of epistemology, where they seem to justify our methods, will first have to be brought closer and adapted to the work of investigating concrete reality.

In the epistemological work of recent years it was particularly emphasized that the task of science is not merely the search for general laws and averages, after the model of the inorganic sciences; there is also the task of describing individuals and types, of which the individual is, after all, merely the limiting case. Windelband and Rickert, by emphasizing this and protesting against the often misleading habits of thought engendered by the physical and chemical sciences, have indeed performed a great service for philosophy. The recognition of these principles has its root in empirical science in so far as it originated in the accurate intuition of a group of people who were at home among the methods of the mental sciences. But these principles received their

logical and scientific justification by methods far removed
from those used in the investigation of facts. They were
not justified by demonstrating the fact that certain aspects
of reality, particularly the psychological, demand a procedure
quite different to that of the inorganic sciences. Nor was the
attempt to justify them made by references to the objects
of investigation and their peculiarities, but by reference to
the transcendental logic of the Kantian schools, which seeks
to determine scientific method from the properties and
demands of our logical, scientific consciousness, and not from
those of the objective world.

The necessity for investigating the individual as well as
the typical was therefore deduced on the basis of the following
considerations : the conceptual system of the natural sciences
continually tends towards greater abstraction and the final
resolution into analytical mechanics, and thus gets further
and further removed from concrete reality. But, like all
thought, scientific thinking is guided by values; and one of
the values it recognizes is that of the apprehension of concrete
reality. But since the natural sciences in their generalizing
procedure are not guided by this particular standpoint of
values, but by its very opposite, there is room for a method
that attempts to apprehend individual, singular, concrete
reality. It does not, therefore, depend on the object and on
the sphere of reality to which it belongs, whether the generalizing or the individualizing method is used, but on what particular value is thought to underlie any research. Both
methods are applicable to the natural and the mental spheres.
According to this view, the objects of the mental world do
not in themselves *demand* the individualizing (or the relatively
individualizing, typological) method ; they can be investigated
by the generalizing method, and this leads to psychology in

the modern sense, which, like any other science, tends towards the final resolution of everything into mechanics. It is true that science as a whole takes greater notice of individual mentality than it does of individual objects in nature ; hence the generalizing method has a closer relation to natural reality, while the individualizing method is more closely related to spiritual reality. But, it is argued, this is not due to the fact that these two levels of reality have a different structure and would therefore need different methods. That the individualizing method is so widely used in the mental sciences is simply due to the fact that in them the standpoint of values is different to that which guides the psychologist, who must use the strict generalizing method.

Now the investigations that are described in this book are psychological ones, and no standpoint has been taken up with regard to the question of values other than that which usually leads to psychology. It was found that the generalizing method had to be partially abandoned and replaced by typological, that is to a certain extent individualizing, methods. This shows clearly that it is above all the *nature* of the subject investigated, the peculiarity of the mental level of reality, which necessitates this change of method. That the exponents of the philosophical sciences made use of the individualizing, or relatively individualizing, method to such a large extent, is not so much due to the fact [1] that their basis of values differs from that of the psychologist, but to the circumstance that with certain intuition, although without conscious reflection, they adapted their method to mental reality.

[1] To a certain extent it is due to this fact as well. But the discussion of this standpoint, to which the investigations of Windelband and Rickert in reality seem to lead, must be reserved for another book.

These questions of method had to be touched upon before, when it was necessary to justify the method of typological investigation. Above all, it seemed necessary to hold this enquiry, in order to counter certain criticisms that were advanced against the eidetic investigations at the outset and that even to-day seem occasionally to be held against them by certain pedagogues. It was objected that investigations of a certain peculiarity in children, which in its most pronounced form was by no means found everywhere, were used to establish *general* conclusions about the development of perceptions and the mentality of youth, and even as a basis for the investigation of wide fields of psychology. To begin with, these conclusions were drawn on the basis of certain pronounced cases. Since such cases are not found very often, if the material is taken from any school not specially selected according to the point of view set out above, it was believed that the eidetic investigations merely treated a special case, which had no general significance for the psychology of childhood and less still for general psychology. But to think this would be to misunderstand entirely the significance of eidetic investigations.

Although our investigations are carried out chiefly on strongly pronounced cases, which, after all, only form the smaller percentage, they nevertheless have a general validity. But it is general validity in a special psychological sense, which differs widely in certain respects from the meaning attached to ' general validity ' in the inorganic sciences. It does not mean here, as in physics or chemistry, that any object of the same species can be substituted for the one that has been examined, just as the chemical analysis of a quantity of mineral water holds true of any other quantity of the same water. The term ' general validity ' as used here has a different, or more accurately, a compound sense :

(1) The characteristics that have been found in the exaggerated cases are only to be found among the average ones in a weaker form. The results of the analyses of pronounced cases will therefore also hold for the weaker cases, if one imagines the strength of all the phenomena to be diminished. But the analysis can only be carried out in all directions by means of the pronounced cases ; therefore it must start from them. That the eidetic investigations have general validity in this sense has been proved by the fact that rudimentary forms of the eidetic faculty could be shown to exist in most, and probably in all children.[1]

(2) The particular characteristic, for whose investigation certain cases were selected in the first instance, is related to other groups of characteristics and structures in the personality, which are also found in the majority of ' average ' cases. It therefore merely serves as a particularly clear index of these other structures. The eidetic faculty, whether it is manifest or merely rudimentary, is an exceptionally clear index of the great importance that sensory experiences have in the life of children. This, again, is the result of a structure of personality, which also seems to be generally prevalent, whose basic property we have called ' coherence ' (*Kohärenz*), *i.e.* the closer intermingling of inner and environmental experiences, and stronger ' integration ' (*Integration*), *i.e.*

---

[1] This result has been verified by the investigations of S. Fischer and Hirschberg, which were carried out in the psychiatric clinic in Breslau. (" Die Verbreitung der eidetischen Anlage im Jugendalter," *Zeitschr. f. d. ges. Neurol. u. Psychiatrie*, 88, 1924). The authors' criticism of the somatic characterization of the types given by W. Jaensch, is due to the fact that they based their research on a " short preliminary note," which did not treat the subject exhaustively. Cf. the monograph by W. Jaensch, *Zur Physiologie und Klinik der psychophysischen Persönlichkeit*, Berlin, 1926.

stronger mutual interpenetration of all psychological functions whatever. The eidetic images are merely a particularly
evident symptom (*stigma*) of these characteristics. For,
when these images are more or less closely related to ideas
(memory images), being at the same time actually *visible*,
the inner and outer experiences of ideation and perception
are in a condition of ' coherence,' and functions that otherwise are separate, are in a condition of mutual interpenetration
or ' integration.' But the same thing is true in children far
beyond this particular phenomenon of eidetic images.

(3) The eidetic investigations can claim general validity
in a third, logically more perfect, sense. It is found that in
the pronounced cases from which we started a certain attribute
of youth is allowed free play. This attribute is also possessed
by the other (weaker) cases ; but, owing to a series of circumstances, it has become atrophied through being starved and
prevented from expressing itself. Wherever the factors
hindering its development have been removed, this attribute
is widely present and even occurs in every individual. The
general validity of eidetic investigations is proved in particular by the fact that the eidetic faculty is extremely
common in children that are being educated according to
the principles of the *Arbeitsschule*. It has further been
shown that the eidetic functional levels are present as dispositions in adults, who otherwise show no signs of eidetic
imagery. Under certain special conditions, *e.g.* when the
subject is very tired after a period of training for sport, these
dispositions may become active.[1]

---

[1] Cf. the investigations of sports from the medical and psychological
sides, on the occasion of the German Academic Olympiad in Marburg, 1924,
particularly the article by E. R. and W. Jaensch. (Published by G. Fischer,
Jena, 1925.)

This threefold sense of 'general validity' is thus seen to be a series of steps. As we go from the first to the third we gradually approximate to the sense in which the term is used in the inorganic sciences, although the two senses never correspond entirely.

We ourselves entered on typological research with some hesitation, just as anyone else will, who has schooled his thinking in the inorganic sciences; nevertheless, it has since justified itself in regions far beyond eidetics.[1] Again, progress can be made in the psychology of later youth, whose important aspects lie in quite different directions to those of eidetic images, if one takes as a starting-point not the phenomena that are immediately evident in *every* individual, but special cases. These may at first sight seem to those not intimately acquainted with the subject to be mere rarities or freaks; but a closer investigation shows that they only present certain general characteristics of this age in an exaggerated form, in 'high relief,' as it were. Recently we have not hesitated to tackle the analysis of a generally prevalent function like abstract thinking[2] from a consideration of certain special cases, which at first sight might be thought to be rarities. But again it was found that these investigations had general validity in the above senses.

We have indicated that the above-mentioned methods are applicable not only in psychology, but apparently in many other branches of the biological sciences. This will be the case wherever these sciences cannot be advanced by the application of methods drawn solely from the inorganic sciences, however valuable these will always be. Indeed the

---

[1] Cf. Part III, below.

[2] *Das unanschauliche Denken, i.e.* thinking that is unaccompanied by visual "images." [Trans.]

same procedure that has been outlined above is also used in investigations of the psychophysical constitution, which have grown out of the eidetic researches. The same *logical* properties, which differ from the methods of the inorganic natural sciences, secure scientific fruitfulness both to eidetics and to researches on the bodily constitution; but at the same time they still seem somewhat strange and unaccustomed to some workers in these fields, and therefore occasionally give rise to misconceptions.

Our procedure in eidetics, in the psychology of childhood and in wide fields of general psychology, consists in attempting to clear up the broad mass of youthful cases by starting with a few special cases to guide us. These special cases have certain characteristics in an exaggerated form, which stick out above the mass, as it were, and are easily discernible. In that way the apparently chaotic and diffuse picture presented by the mass can be made clear.

Medical men have also for some time past been interested in a certain broad group of youthful persons within the larger mass—not counting those suffering from specific diseases, in whom they have always been interested. This is the group variously labelled ' nervous,' ' slightly psychopathic,' ' deficient,' or ' anomalous' in various respects, to which should be added the mentally deficient, unintelligent, and the slow thinkers. The subdivisions in this group are not at all clearly marked, and it has therefore often been compared to a drawer, in which all that is put, to which no definite, fixed place can be assigned. In spite of numerous attempts it has not seemed possible hitherto to analyse this group from within, that is, by starting investigations from the group itself, just as the far wider group of childhood as such could not be analysed and interpreted from itself, as far as certain fundamental characteristics were concerned. As long as we choose our standpoint within the group, these youthful neuropaths and psychopaths present a chaotic picture, with no clear lines for orientation. But we can bring clearness into the chaotic picture of the psychology of child-hood, by starting with cases in which normal characteristics are present in an exaggerated form ; the same applies here. Here, too, greater transparency is only brought about in our initially chaotic picture when we take up our standpoint outside the general mass to begin with, and start with cases that stand up out of the general mass. These cases will naturally approach the region of definite disease and belong to well-defined clinical disease pictures. In the broad mass of different ' deficients ' we shall then be able to trace the origins and rudiments or merely hardly noticeable indications of those phenomena, which, in our special cases, were seen in the strong light of exaggeration. It is then easy to follow downwards the sharp lines given by these cases that stand out from the mass, and the chaotic picture will be resolvable into a clear network of intersecting lines that differentiate various forms from one another. Only by the help of this method, whose logical basis is the same as that of the eidetic investigations, was it possible to obtain the following results from the constitutional investigations that grew out of the eidetic ones. These results hope to make possible a far closer co-operation between teacher and doctor than is at present possible. They therefore deserve the interest of all teachers.[1]

---

[1] Cf. Walther Jaensch, lecture delivered to the VII congress for experim. psychology in Marburg, 1921 (*Bericht ü. d. VII Kongr. f. exp. Psych.*, Jena, 1922) ; *Münchener med. Wochenschr.*, Nr. 35, 1921 ; *Monatsschr. f. Kinderheilk*, 1921 ; W. Jaensch und W. Wittneben, *Zeitschr. f. Kinder-forschung*, 1924, in their report on the *Kongress für Heilpädagogik*, Munich, 1924.

It was mentioned above that the normal B-type, whose exaggerated form has Graves' or Basedow's disease, is so common in youth that it must be looked upon as one of the normal characteristics of the age before puberty. As is well known, the pathological form of this normal youthful stigma, Graves' disease, is connected with an increased functioning of the thyroid gland, *i.e.* hyperthyreosis. Teachers will know that school children very often show a slight swelling of the thyroid gland, known as ' school goitre.' Since the phenomenon of hyperthyreosis is so common in youth, the question arose whether its opposite, hypothyreosis, was at all common in normal persons. As has long been known, a subnormal functioning of the thyroid gland leads to myxœdema, which is recognized by certain changes, above all by a thickening of the skin, together with a general slowing down and obstruction of all mental functions. According to the gravity of the case, this may lead to various forms of mental deficiency. Innate myxœdema in early childhood, which is occasionally due to absence of the thyroid gland (athyreosis), is further accompanied by serious disturbances of growth and the retention of infantile stages both mentally and in various organs, such as the retention of down and milk teeth. Non-innate myxœdema, unless induced by an operation, is a very rare disease.

In most cases it can be successfully influenced by feeding with animal thyroid extracts. As a rule this even cures the disease, removing both physical and mental symptoms, at any rate while the thyroid feeding is continued. Even in innate myxœdema and athyreosis great improvements and an acceleration of development up to an approximately normal level are possible if the treatment begins early enough.[1] The best results are naturally achieved if the treatment is begun in the sibling. Unfortunately even the most pronounced cases of this kind are generally only noticed when the best time for treatment has passed. The question arises, therefore, whether there exists a normal psychophysical constitution related to myxœdema in a similar way in which the B-type is related to Basedow's disease, that is, a type whose pathological exaggeration is myxœdema.

It became necessary to search for rudimentary symptoms of myxœdematism and to work out more delicate methods, which would be able to register such rudimentary symptoms. It happened by good fortune that W. Jaensch examined the skin capillaries of a hypothyroidic cretin in the medical clinic at Marburg (which was at that time directed by G. von Bergmann). This method, which had been introduced into the technique of clinical examination in the Tübingen clinic (Otfried Müller, E. Weiss), enables one to make a simple and easy microscopic examination of the structure and function of the finest cutaneous vessels at the base of the nail in a living subject.[2] This spot, where the skin grows over the nail, is particularly suited to such an examination, since the capillaries are parallel to the surface, not, as is usual, perpendicular. They can therefore be investigated for some distance along their course. Normally,

---

[1] The form of hypothyreosis, accompanied by distinct symptoms of myxœdema, which occurs endemically in certain regions (*e.g.* in the Schwund district of Styria), is an exception. It is usually called 'cretinism,' but a better term would perhaps be 'true hypothyroidic cretinism.' Even when the treatment is extended over many years, only a low level of development is achieved. This refractory behaviour of cretinism towards thyroid therapy (within certain limits) has recently been attributed by Finkbeiner to local (endemic) blood admixture of primitive races.

[2] Cf. Walther Jaensch, *Die Hautkapillarmikroskopie*, Halle, 1929.

these capillaries have the form of hairpins. Arterial and venous blood meet, each forming one shank of the ' hairpin.' The capillaries come out of the *rete subpapillare*, which is perpendicular to them. In the case of this hypothyroidic cretin the conditions were very different from the normal. Instead of the forms having a normal hairpin shape, they were much more irregular, drawn apart laterally, and could only be compared to a vine tendril or a knocker. Since changes in the skin are characteristic of the myxœdemic condition, and since a particularly delicate method was at hand, which had led to a remarkable discovery in an authentic case of hypothyreosis, it seemed worth while using this delicate test to find out whether there was a parallel to this hypothyroidic symptom outside actually diseased cases. Since the hypothyroidic condition is accompanied by more or less serious mental retardation, it was expected that if such cases existed at all, they would most likely be found among pupils of *Hilfsschulen* (schools for mentally deficient children).

In the very first class of backward children to be investigated in Marburg by means of the capillary test the great majority of pupils showed conditions, which deviated from the norm in exactly the same way, though less strongly, as did those of the myxœdemic cretin. On the other hand, a control investigation carried out in a class of normal children, showed that the great majority had normal hairpin forms. During the last few years these results have been verified over and again in different places. The preliminary results showed, and later researches have verified, that this method places at our disposal the means of differentiating between various forms of mental inferiority. These cases of backwardness have not only the qualitative criterion of similar capillaries in common with myxœdemic cretinism ; in both cases they are the result of general physical and mental arrested development. They must therefore be classified among the so-called ' infantilisms,' and in the less pronounced cases they are most quickly and easily discernible by means of the capillary test. This test is therefore one of the most delicate reagents for such conditions, and it is as such that it acquires its importance.

Even more important than the recognition of certain forms of feeble-mindedness and the indication of their therapy, is the correct diagnosis of the origin of certain neuropathic diseases, which is possible by means of this test. The degenerative variants of the capillaries found in such cases are probably only partially due to anharmonic differentiation during development. Myxœdemic cretinism is the ultimate result of a faulty balance of the inner secretions, which is also present in the milder cases. The cases of pupils in these *Hilfsschulen* that do not show the abnormal capillaries, however, are due to other causes, such as damage done by environment or education, luetic or alcoholic degeneration, etc. In the *Hilfsschulen* of Marburg, Cassel, and Heidelberg, the cases with strongly divergent capillaries are in the majority. These towns all lie in so-called ' goitre districts.' But in the schools of Frankfurt, which is free from goitre, cases in which the capillaries are normal are in the majority ; in fact, they are almost the rule, which is only occasionally broken by a case with degenerate capillaries. As a rule the subjects with degenerate capillaries found in goitre regions have a lower average intelligence than the subjects in schools where the capillaries are normal, and where the feeble-mindedness is therefore due to other causes. This accounts for an observation that has often been made

by the teachers of the province of Hesse-Nassau, that quite
different demands have to be made in the *Hilfsschulen*
of Cassel and Frankfurt and that therefore different curricula
are necessary.   In the schools of small towns and villages
in districts that are particularly prone to such developmental arrest, the backward children are not removed to
special schools, but mingle with the other children.   In
such schools it may happen that a class has such a large
proportion of pupils who show capillary arrest, that they
depress the level of the class, increase the difficulties of the
teacher and retard the progress of normal pupils.   In certain
goitre regions, as in some villages of the Badenese Neckar
valley [1] (*e.g.*, in Dilsberg near Neckarsteinach) the average
capillary finding of a normal class may reveal a greater
developmental arrest than is found in the *Hilfsschulen* of
other regions, even goitre regions, not to mention the
Hilfsschulen of regions free from goitre.   In other small
villages within a goitre region (*e.g.*, in Marbach near Marburg),
the capillary findings in a normal class still show a greater
divergence than in the *Hilfsschulen* of Frankfurt, which is
free from goitre.   This explains the assertion which teachers
in such schools have often made, that, although they are
supposed to be teaching a ' normal ' class, they have the
feeling of being in a *Hilfsschule*.   It follows from this, that
the curricula ought to take account of such local differences,
and that it is unjustifiable to make the same demands of
teachers in such districts as Hesse-Nassau without taking
them into account, and merely differentiating between
' normal ' schools and *Hilfsschulen*.   Many contradictions

---

[1] Our best thanks are due to the psychiatric clinic in Heidelberg, particularly to its director, Professor Wilmanns, for making these investigations
possible.

between the keenness and capacity of a teacher, and the actual results achieved, is explained by these facts, as well as many observations of local differences, which may have been made intuitively by teachers or officials of the education departments, who had no accurate criteria. The fact that the divergent capillary forms of goitre regions are also to be found in normal schools in which no backward children have been segregated, is due to the fact that the developmental arrest which underlies them occurs endemically in wide regions. Such occasional findings among pupils of normal schools do not, therefore, alter the fact that fully intelligent pupils who are not neuropathic, everywhere show normal capillaries. If the intelligence is normal and the capillaries nevertheless show a greater degree of abnormality, it always points to a neuro-pathological case caused by a partial developmental arrest, that is, a disharmonic development. According to its localization and the type of personality, this will have different characteristics. But this type of arrested development must not be thought to be the same as or due to ' school goitre ' ; even in classes where it is prevalent school goitre may be entirely absent. The developmental arrest, whose stigma is abnormal capillaries, does not start in the later years of childhood, as school goitre is assumed to do ; it is due to very early childish conditions of the vascular systems in the skin being retained and with them, probably, conditions in the central nervous system that are connected with them. This is shown by the investigation of capillary development during the first weeks after birth of the normal infant. In regions free from goitre this development is completed by the end of the first year ; in goitre regions it often seems to progress much more slowly. The abnormal capillary forms, which prove to be characteristic for those arrests in development, simply arise because various levels of capillary development are retained without the development being concluded. A phylogenetic parallel to this developmental arrest, which shows itself in the preservation of the vascular systems of early childhood, has already been discovered. Subject to further research, we can already say that adults of the higher vertebrates have the capillary forms that appear last in the human child, whilst the lower vertebrates only have the early, least differentiated, capillary forms.

The abnormal capillaries that are characteristic of the arrested development discussed above, were first observed in a case of myxœdemic cretinism and were later found to be a regular concomitant of cretinism. With respect to the capillaries there is thus a connection between the arrest of development in question and conditions like that of myxœdema, in which there is a loss of function or even a total absence of the thyroid gland. It is known that arrested development caused by myxœdema in early childhood can be compensated for to a very large extent by feeding with animal thyroid extract. Successful treatment of our true cretinic material went parallel with a gradual further differentiation of the capillaries. Thyroid feeding was therefore tried on those cases of arrested development that did not belong to the class of myxœdemic cretinism, but that had the capillary abnormalities in common with it. It was found that these cases, too, respond with progress in growth and intellectual development as well as with increased differentiation of the capillaries. Those cases whose capillary development was more backward responded better than the more advanced ones, whilst feeble-minded individuals or those with *normal* capillaries showed no change at all in the control cases that have been treated so far. When there was no change in individuals with marked capillary arrest, it was due, as far as we have been able to determine up to the present, to other factors, such as trauma at birth, hereditary lues, infantile encephalitis or meningitis, or, as the X-ray analysis showed, to changes in the hypophysis, which is also known to determine infantile arrest of development. The disturbance of development of hypophyseal origin, which often shows itself only in the arrest of the capillaries, does not necessarily show any of the symptoms that have hitherto been regarded as evidence of this very rare hypophyseal disturbance. Nevertheless, arrested development due to such disturbances responds to feeding of animal hypophysis extract, in the cases that have come under our observation. The above remarks all seem to hold true of individuals with widely different neuropathic symptoms who have arrested capillaries.[1]

Arrested development is very common, even endemic, in certain parts. It therefore seemed advisable to try whether similar therapeutic success could not be achieved with simpler and cheaper methods, which could be applied more generally. It was shown by extensive treatment that minimal doses of iodine salts were in the long run equivalent to thyroid extracts, except perhaps in the cases of hypophyseal origin and those in which there is an obvious gross disturbance of the function of some particular gland, as in true myxœdema. If the cases are still capable of develop-

---

[1] The first experiments of W. Jaensch were carried out in Marburg with the help of Mr Buisman ; further experiments in *Hilfsschule* II in Cassel, with the help of the principal, Mr Gonnermann, Miss Nennstiehl, and Dr Scholl. Extensive series were then carried out by W. Jaensch in the Hephata asylum near Treysa, Cassel, in conjunction with the medical director, Dr Wittneben.

ment, they are on the whole improved ; the others are not harmed by the treatment.

It seems possible, therefore, that a systematic prophylactic, similar to goitre prophylactic in Switzerland, might decrease the number of backward children in the endemic areas, provided iodine treatment begins early enough and not as late as the compulsory school age, as is the case in goitre prophylactic in the south of Germany. This prophylactic, which could be achieved by adding small quantities of iodine to the common salt sold to the populace, as in Switzerland, would have to start before birth. But a prophylactic of this kind has hitherto been rejected as being superfluous by the exponents of school goitre prophylactic in south Germany, on the grounds that, except for sporadic cases, goitre in Germany is not accompanied by a general distribution of cretinism as in Switzerland. But it has been shown that, although pure cases of cretinism are not very frequent in the German goitre regions, other types of arrested development occur, which have capillary arrest in common with cretinism and together with it belong to the large group of infantile feeble-mindedness, or infantilisms in general. In regions such as these, where there is no endemic cretinism as in Switzerland, only endemic arrested development, the conditions for a successful general prophylactic are particularly favourable, much more favourable than in regions with endemic cretinism, which is assumed to have a quite different root—blood admixture of primitive alien races—and this is naturally not accessible to prophylactic. If this type of general prophylactic is continued for a number of generations, we should expect that the level of bodily and mental development of whole populaces would be raised.

It will take some time before these points of view are generally appreciated. The difficulty in the way is the same as that which long prevented a proper understanding of eidetics, and even to-day prevents it in some cases : the lack of appreciation of the importance of the typological method. To the representatives of the sciences of mental life (*Geisteswissenschaften*), particularly since Dilthey, this method is well known ; but to the psychologist, natural scientist and medical man it still seems strange and unfamiliar. The way in which the typological method obtains results that are subsequently shown to be valid for the average mass, is not along the shortest and most direct route. The nearest way of discovering general principles which has hitherto been followed, consists in starting out from that which can be observed in the average case, that is, which in principle could be done by means of a statistical enquiry, if only the enquiry could be accurate enough for each case. The typological method has quite a different starting-point, although it, too, eventually leads to the normal average case. It starts by seeking the connection between this normal average and certain special cases that emerge out of the undifferentiated average level in a certain way. It then tries to interpret this average level from the light thrown on it by these special cases.

This method has to face two different but equally strong prejudices and obstructions among investigators in the biological sciences. The ' normal ' psychologist and the teacher point out that they are concerned with the normal, the average, that which can in principle always be arrived at by means of a mass-enquiry. They are prone to regarding it as a wilful caprice to be asked to start their investigation of normality with cases that do not quite conform to it.

For a similar reason the attitude of medical men is not very favourable towards the typological method of connecting true clinical cases with cases that are still normal. We have experienced over and again that in some cases it is almost impossible to lead them to attend to non-clinical material and the differences that exist there. They merely say that these differences ' are of no importance,' simply because they do not happen to be ' pathological ' or to fit into well-known syndroma. The significance of the typological method is realized most strongly at the present time among those students of life,[1] who have freed themselves of the habits of thought inculcated by the inorganic sciences; in the sciences of the highest manifestations of mental life, culture and history.[2]

J. von Kries has always been foremost in recognizing that the progress of science depends in a great measure on the further development and elucidation of our logical methods and forms of thinking. In the times of Galileo, Descartes and Leibniz, the development of the forms of thought adapted to those of inorganic nature did not proceed by means of an epistemology divorced from individual research, but by an epistemology that grew in intimate contact with it. So to-day only a direction of research that carries out the logical elucidation of method, together with work on the object itself, will be able to advance those branches of the biological sciences that are some distance removed from the inorganic sciences. This is not meant

---

[1] Among psychologists the methods advocated here were first seriously considered by the few investigators like G. Störring, who hoped to gain insight into normal psychology from a study of psychopathological phenomena. The pronounced types, which are still within the normal range, are the most important.

[2] Cf. Part II.

as a pretentious analogy, intended to make the problems that are the particular care of our generation appear to have universal importance. It is merely meant to indicate that the intimate co-operation of logical thought and individual research is as necessary to-day as it was then. That is why we have attempted to present a few of the main results of our work, with particular reference to the logical and methodological aspects that have guided the majority of our scientific efforts.

PART II

AFTER what has been said about psychological methods above, it will be understood why a leading psychiatrist, O. Bumke, believes that he can find more points of contact with the ' humanistic ' psychology of E. Spranger, who is of the Dilthey school, than with experimental psychology, which, he thinks, has reached the limits of its usefulness.[2] The psychiatrist, like the exponent of ' humanistic ' psychology, is always concerned with an individual *as a whole*, and with different human *types*, which emerge under such a treatment. Certain deficiencies of experimental psychology, which clung to it in the beginning when its methods were still to a large extent modelled on those of the inorganic sciences, would therefore be noticed most by him. Such deficiencies, from his

---

[1] ' *Naturwissenschaftliche* ' *und* ' *geisteswissenschaftliche* ' *Psychologie.*

[2] O. Bumke, " Psychologie und Psychiatrie," *Klinische Wochenschrift.* 1922.—Postscript : While reading this essay for the last time, I had an opportunity of discussing these questions with Geheimrat Bumke. Our views were in complete agreement. O. Bumke repudiates most strongly any assertion that he is antagonistic to experimental psychology. But he shares our view that through having been occupied for too long with psychophysics, and remaining attached in too one-sided a fashion to a purely physical point of view, psychology has not really touched upon the questions of the inner psychic life. It has therefore fulfilled only a very small part of the hopes, which psychiatry had placed on it. Now it is precisely our view that it is not permissible to transpose the methods of physics into psychology without adaptation, and our ' typological method ' is an attempt to make this necessary adaptation. In these pages we have tried to present this method, which enables us to bridge the gulf between naturalistic, experimental psychology and humanistic psychology.

point of view, would be the 'prejudice of uniformity,' which overlooked all typical differences; the lack of any tendency to take account of the *whole* personality; the over-emphasis of the physiology of the senses; the 'physicalism' of overhastily drawn-up theories, whose ideal seemed at one time to be a mechanics of psychic elements; the 'intellectualism' of these theories, which only takes account of those aspects of psychic events that are most amenable to such 'physicalistic' treatment, and in doing so overlooks those aspects of personality, which seem to the psychiatrist and to the humanistic psychologist the ones that really determine psychic events, and therefore the most important. Although we must admit these objections, as far as they are concerned with the initial stages of our science, we must, nevertheless, bear in mind the following in defence of the psychology which starts from the side of the natural sciences : these objections are no longer wholly true in respect of the psychology of the present day. We know for certain that Spranger himself is convinced that the time has passed in which the two forms of psychology are strictly opposed to one another, and that a closer co-operation is being established. As a matter of fact some psychiatrists occasionally advise psychology to proceed in precisely the opposite direction, to work even more strictly and exclusively as a natural science. Only then, they think, will its service to the more clinical branches of science become clearly visible. Thus Bleuler, the master of schizophrenic research, once wrote me a very temperamental letter to the effect that the psychological researches being carried out here were " pure natural science "; we ought fully to admit this and keep them strictly free from philosophic or humanistic (*geisteswissenschaftliche*) lines of thought, which had for so long prevented the development of psychology into a science.

In our work we have always sought contact with the natural as well as with the philosophical sciences and have found that this attitude has proved its worth. In the above-mentioned article Bumke also criticizes the attempts that are occasionally made nowadays to place psychiatry on a purely *geisteswissenschaftliche* foundation (in the sense of Husserl's so-called ' phenomenology '). But Bumke's remarks about the necessity that the standpoint in psychiatry should at the same time be that of the natural sciences, apply equally well to psychology. In spite of the attitude taken over from the natural sciences, psychology need not forgo its attempt to take account of the whole personality. Any experimental procedure must necessarily apply a lever to the analysis of some particular individual function. But this procedure does not include the assertion that the functional parts, which for reasons of method have been isolated, form the whole being merely summatively, without being mutually interrelated, as independent grains of sand together make up a heap. A functional part can serve as the point of application of the method by means of which the psychologist reaches the interpretation of the whole being and his characteristic type, just as the psychology of everyday life always starts from single points or impressions.[1]

[1] This tendency to apprehend the *whole* is not merely a characteristic of everyday psychology, which Bumke opposes to experimental psychology, but a necessary property of *every* science that tries to reach a deeper conception of its subject. Theoretical physics, general and comparative physiology, the general history of culture and thought and many other branches of knowledge actually owe their existence to this tendency. The fact that experimental psychology for some time did not include this point of view is not due to its being a *cul-de-sac*, but to the general position of science at the time in which it began. Soon after psychology had taken its first steps, the phase of positivism set in, and because of this, ' wholes '

According to the measure in which psychology is *also* orientated towards the natural sciences and uses experimental data, it will reach a more complete, richer and in many respects deeper view of the total personality and of human types than everyday psychology. Furthermore, the psychology that is allied to the natural sciences, however closely it may approach philosophic methods, will always insist on a rigorously *empirical* procedure, which bases all its conclusions only on observations and facts. It will therefore need to exercise restraint in using many of the methods that *geisteswissenschaftliche* psychology has developed because of its origin in the sciences of history and culture. The conclusions of psychology will therefore at first also avoid establishing a close contact with cultural values and will not immediately attempt to combine methodically the observation of empirical facts with the establishment of norms and values. Nevertheless, although psychology may

were pushed into the background in all the sciences, both natural and philosophic. This phase of development has passed ; we can still thankfully retain the valuable things this period produced, without retaining its undeniably narrow point of view. Where this point of view has been superseded and the tendency towards the apprehension of wholes is again to the fore, most of the older sciences will be able to look back to a tradition in this direction, which was only broken during the relatively short rule of positivism. Scientific psychology is in a less favourable position in this respect, since the short period in which it has been in existence fell almost entirely within the period of positivism. (We need not emphasize, however, that psychology is not a *product* of positivism and positivistic modes of thinking.) For this reason new starting-points for research have to be uncovered in psychology more than in any other science, if the tendency towards wholes, which is so noticeable in other sciences, is to come into its own in psychology as well. But these starting-points are present and are daily leading us further.

This question is also treated in our article in *Kantstudien*, " Zum Gedächtnis von Alois Riehl," in which the attempt is made to trace the general results of positivism in the sciences. The peculiar position of psychology is nowhere mentioned, but because psychology is connected with the general attitude of the time, an analysis of that attitude will also provide us with the material for judging various psychological currents.

exercise restraint with regard to questions of value and norm during the process of research, this does not exclude the possibility that it may be able to make valuable contributions to these questions in spite of, or rather because of its attitude towards the discovery of facts. This will be the case when experimental methods bring to light aspects of human life, which have hitherto, or at any rate in the civilization in which we live, not been sufficiently taken into account, and which could be made to serve the progress of mental development by being more strongly emphasized.

PART III

Recent Developments in Eidetics, with particular
reference to the General Psychology of the
Senses and to Typology

I HAVE much pleasure in adding a few words on recent developments to the English edition of the *Eidetik*, which my pupil and friend, Oscar Oeser, has prepared.

The first edition of this small book has been far better received than I hoped or expected. In particular it has brought me many external collaborators. In testimony of this there are the numerous publications on eidetic imagery, which every month continue to swell the already large volume of literature on the subject. " *Die Sache ist in Fluss gekommen*," as the German has it. I could have included all the recent publications in the body of this English edition. But even then only a particular phase would have been described ; and to-morrow that will have been replaced by a new one. I have therefore preferred to leave the book in the form in which it has had its influence on science and in which it has become a part of science. But I wish to indicate here the general directions that this work has taken in psychological, medical, and philosophic fields.

I have always been of opinion that the growth of science takes place chiefly in the fields that lie along the dividing line between one science and another, and I have therefore always had a predilection for working at problems in which several branches of investigation overlap. Eidetics are an outstanding example of this kind of work. I am well aware of the fact that in England psychology is treated far more as a special science than is the case in Germany. But I would ask the English reader not to be alarmed if the general work that started from eidetics has also led us to consider some general philosophical problems, and in this English edition I least of all wish to omit all mention of these. The firm footing that English thinking in particular has in experience, is of the utmost value for philosophy, and should never be abandoned. Cartesianism, which has always been inimical to experience, still dominates wide fields of psychology and particularly philosophy.[1] Empirical thinking (*Wirklichkeitsdenken*) and the standpoint of experience have to fight hard to prevail; and in this fight nothing has strengthened me more than the works of the great leaders of English philosophy. To Bacon and Hobbes, to Locke as well as to Hume, the problems of philosophy were empirical, and largely to be solved by the methods of psychology. It is an urgent need, not only of science, but of civilization and of life, that this task should once more be seen in this light, and that psychology should receive the recognition that is its due.

Psychology, which can say of itself *nihil humani mihi est alienum*, is particularly close to life. If the problems of civilization and of life are faced from an empirical, instead of an *a priori* standpoint, psychology will have an important part to play. While our book *Grundformen menschlichen Seins* (published by O. Elsner, Berlin, 1930), was in the press, our great political leader Stresemann died. To point

---

[1] Cf. our essay, "Der latente Cartesianismus der modernen Wissenschaft," in the 16. *Ergänzungsband, Zeitschr. f. Psychologie*, 1930.

out more clearly the importance of psychology for the problems of life, I added a short chapter to the already completed work, which gives a psychological characterization of Stresemann and tries to prove the importance of psychology in the relationships of nations. After what has been said above, I need not discuss further how much I expect of a close co-operation between England and Germany with regard to this standpoint of empirical thinking and experience.

Let us return to the development of eidetics. Of the investigations that have come from other centres than Marburg, those of Bonte and Rössler seem to me particularly helpful.[1] Eidetic phenomena could not lay claim to any general interest, if, as has occasionally been alleged, they are in every one of their forms symptoms of a lower grade of intelligence. Bonte's proof that that is not the case, is in accord with our own work.[2] Other investigations have been directed towards discovering the age at which eidetic phenomena are most widely prevalent.

Eidetic phenomena are of great importance because the mental structures manifesting themselves in them are intimately concerned with the building up of the perceptual world. Since this development must take place in early youth, there could be no justification for postulating such a connection if, as some authors have supposed, eidetic phenomena occur only in *later* youth, *e.g.* just before puberty. We ourselves have not in general started earlier than the tenth year, since it is difficult to work with still younger subjects. But as a result of our observations we have

---

[1] Bonte und Rössler, *Beihefte zur Zeitschr. für angew. Psychol.*, 43, 1928.
[2] Cf. Karoline Schmitz, " Über das anschauliche Denken und die Frage einer Korrelation zwischen eidetischer Anlage und Intelligenz," *Zeitschr. f. Psychol.*, 114, 1930.

always been of opinion that the frequency of eidetic phenomena is higher in younger children, and that a much higher
percentage would be found, if younger children could be
tested with the same accuracy as older ones. Rössler has
very cleverly overcome the difficulties that stand in the
way of eidetic investigations with young children. He
found the maximum disposition for having eidetic images
in the youngest class examined by him, the sixth year.
The same result was reached in an investigation carried out
on after-images in my institute by J. Gross.[1] Since the
eidetic images are intermediate between after-images and
memory images, the problem can also be attacked from the
side of after-images. It is then possible to find whether
and in how far these after-images differ from those on which
physiology bases its discussions, and whether they have
moved up the scale in the direction of memory images.
One tries to find out in how far after-images are coupled
to the sphere of memory images, that is, to what degree
sensations are interrelated with ideas. In terms of our
typology this means determining to what extent the individual shows ' integration,' which is one of the characteristics
of youth. The results obtained by Gross were in agreement
with those of Rössler, who had worked quite independently
of us. They showed that the integration of after-image
and memory image, and with it the latent eidetic disposition,
was at a maximum in early childhood ; but this is the age
at which the perceptual world is being built up. Thus one
of the main arguments against our theory of the development
of perceptions has been met.

---

[1] J. Gross, " Experimentaluntersuchungen über den Integrationsgrad bei
Kindern," *Zeitschr. f. angew. Psychol.*, Vol. 33, 1929, reprinted in *Studien
zur Psychologie Menschlicher Typen*, Leipzig, 1930.

This theory has been set forth in two monographs from two different, but complementary points of view. In " *Über den Aufbau der Wahrnehmungswelt* " (second edition, Leipzig, 1927) it was shown that the perceptual world of children and adult eidetic subjects differed from that of the average adult. The behaviour of eidetic phenomena was compared to that of the perception of real objects. It was found that real perceptual objects behaved in a similar fashion to eidetic images, that is, they have been moved along the scale in the direction of eidetic phenomena. This result of extensive experimental investigations can also be expressed as follows : during the eidetic phase of development the perceptual world is ' hemieidetic.' Since eidetic phenomena are intermediate between perceptions and true memory images, this means that the primary perceptions are very close to memory images. In the course of development this peculiarity is gradually lost. Perceptions gradually achieve an ever higher degree of point-to-point correspondence with external stimuli. This development is the exact opposite of that hitherto assumed by the perceptual theories of Helmholtz and Hering, which, although they differ in many respects, are in agreement on this point. For they both think that pure sensations, unaffected by higher mental processes, are the starting-point for development, and that a greater measure of mental assimilation gradually takes place. Actually it is just the other way round : sensations that are permeated with higher mental processes (*Vorstellungen*), form the starting-point for development ; and ' primary ' sensations, *i.e.* sensations that correspond exactly to external stimuli, are the ideal end-point of this development, which is never quite reached. We have shown that this peculiar course of development is in accord with anatomical facts ; anatomically, the eye is originally a cerebral organ. Only later does it become more exclusively an organ for conducting external stimuli, whilst parallel to this development sensations begin to correspond more and more accurately to external stimuli and to depend less on higher mental processes.

This peculiar characteristic of the development of sight is particularly clear in spatial perceptions, but it is also found in colour vision. Here, too, is the key to phenomena that have been much discussed in recent years, the ' approximate constancy of visual objects ' or ' colour transformation,' as is shown in the investigations collected under the title " *Grundfragen der Farbenpsychologie* " (Leipzig, 1930). Our eyes do not see external objects according to the physical state of illumination ; when objects are being perceived the illumination (or the shadow) are, as it were, subtracted. Hitherto there have been two opinions on the matter. The empirical interpretations of Helmholtz and Katz assumed that colour constancy can only be explained through the experience of visual objects having colour constancy, that is, by means of associations. As in the theory of the spatial sense, Hering held a nativistic conception. He rightly pointed out that the empirical explanation is a circular argument. For, in order to gather experiences about visual objects of ' constant colour,' we must already possess the phenomenon of ' approximate colour constancy.' Hering therefore taught that colour constancy is innately bound up with certain functions of the eye. He believed that it can be explained by contrast, pupillary reaction, and above all by adaptation. These processes will, for example, make a disc situated in shadow appear brighter. We have dedicated our own work on this subject to the memory of Ewald

Hering, to give expression to our conviction that the great investigator was on the right track in this respect too. He could not, however, penetrate to the real explanation, because he only worked with adults. But, as in the case of spatial perception, an understanding of the underlying laws can only be reached by genetic methods. The factors by means of which Hering attempts an explanation of colour transformation, are inadequate for two reasons. They are insufficient quantitatively, and, since they only depend on external stimuli, they do not take into account psychological factors, although these are undoubtedly present in the phenomena of colour transformation.

The investigations collected in our monograph, " *Über den Aufbau der Wahrnehmungswelt*," showed that the spatial perceptions were a ' precipitate,' a ' petrifaction ' of those functional factors determining the development of the perceptual world for the individual, and very probably for the species as well. Exactly the same *genetic* methods lead to the goal in the problem of colour transformation. In the early eidetic phase, adaptation actually has the properties it should have in order to explain colour transformation. It is quantitatively higher and, like so many physiological processes in childhood, it is ' psychologically integrated,' that is, it does not depend merely on external stimuli, but on mental factors as well.[1] The close relation to the eidetic facts will become clear, if one keeps in mind the indissoluble connection between after-images and the process of adaptation. If a limited area of the visual field

[1] In addition to the investigations collected in " *Grundfragen der Farbenpsychologie*," the following is important : A. Heinemann, " Über die Dunkeladaptation usw.," *Zeitschr. f. Sinnesphysiol.*, 60 (1929). He shows that the Purkinje phenomenon, which gives a measure of the capacity for adaptation, can be seven times as strong in children who are in the eidetic phase of development, as it is in adults.

is stimulated by a colour, an after-image arises there. If the whole visual field is exposed to the colour, adaptation takes place. *Both* are due to the antagonistic process beginning to function, in the one case in a limited area, in the other over the whole visual field. As eidetics has shown, the former is quantitatively far more pronounced in children who are in the eidetic phase of development, than it is in adults, and it is integrated with the sphere of memory images (*Vorstellungen*), that is, it is dependent on memory images. Hence it is very probable that the same will be true of the process of adaptation, which is so closely connected with the process giving rise to after-images. This is found to be the case. In the monograph " *Aufbau der Wahrnehmungswelt* " we had shown that spatial values are a precipitate or petrifaction of processes that are active in the development of the optical world during the early phases of vision. Conditions are exactly the same in colour vision. The transformation phenomena are a precipitate of processes active during the early phases, and the contrast phenomena have the same origin. This explains the complete *parallelism of laws*, which, as we were able to show experimentally, obtains between contrast and transformation phenomena. The facts are entirely against the purely empirical interpretation, which Katz gave to the phenomena of colour transformation. It can be understood why the attempt should have been made to explain these phenomena purely by means of associations, but contrast cannot be explained in this way. One would then have to explain contrast and transformation in entirely different ways ; but in that case the parallelism between the laws of these two phenomena, which holds down to small details, must remain an unintelligible miracle.

All these facts, particularly the integration with the mental sphere, show that the eye takes up a special position. It is pre-eminently a ' brain organ,' and vision is a sense that is ' psychical ' to a special degree, in that even its elementary functions are integrated with the higher mental sphere. We can understand why the sense of sight has always had so much attention in psychological investigations. These facts also suggest the need for a comparative psychology and physiology of the senses, particularly if our acoustical investigations are taken into account.

We have examined the nature of phonetic sounds by means of the selenium siren, which enables sound curves to be varied at will. It was found that vowels are an intermediate structure between tones and noises. They arise when the average value of successive waves remains close to a certain mean value, although it is the presence of ' disturbing factors,' which differentiates noise curves from a succession of exactly equal waves.[1] If we look at the totality of acoustic and non-acoustic functions of the ear, this organ proves to be a ' seismic sense ' with seismographs, i.e., registering apparatus, of continually increasing delicacy.[2]

The otoliths and the semicircular canals serve the perception of coarse mass movements. The noise sense at any rate can react roughly to differences of pitch ; the vowel sense is an indicator for the average value of successive wavelengths ; the tone sense is an indicator for these wave-

[1] This result only appears strange as long as the ear is thought of as an analytic organ under all circumstances whatever, as Helmholtz conceived it, and that therefore acoustic stimuli should always be thought of from the point of view of Fourier analysis. But the analytic function of the ear does not come into play at all during the hearing of vowels. Hence there is no necessity for Fourier analysis in characterizing the stimuli.

[2] E. R. Jaensch (und Mitarbeiter), *Untersuchungen über Grundfragen der Akustik und Tonpsychologie*, Leipzig, 1929.

lengths themselves. The ' seismic ' character of the ear is in agreement with the fact that it is a cutaneous sense organ ; the completely different structure and function of the eye is due to its being a cerebral organ. That explains why acoustic eidetic phenomena are about ten times rarer than optical ones in children. While eidetic factors are operative in the development of ordinary vision, the development of the acoustic functions takes place without this central (cerebral) intervention. Eidetic factors only come into play in musical hearing, which, according to G. Révész, is based on special musical qualities. Eye and ear are therefore quite different even in respect of eidetic qualities.

But let us first complete the discussion of the development of the perceptual world. We shall now follow the lines of thought set forth in the second monograph dedicated to this subject.[1] The first monograph was based on eidetic subjects, *i.e.*, selected material ; the second is based on unselected youthful observers.

It was shown that the hemieidetic peculiarities in perception, which were plainly evident in eidetic subjects, are present to a greater or lesser degree in all youthful subjects. For example, the definite and monovalent association of the perception of depth with certain values of transverse retinal disparity is a result of individual development. The perceptions of children are in every case nearer to ideas (*Vorstellungen*) and are integrated with the imaginal levels and the total psychic contents. But even in fully differentiated perception, a residue of integration is found to be present, as is shown by the work of F. Simon [2] in the mono-

---

[1] *Über den Aufbau des Bewussseinds*, 16. Ergänzungsband, *Zeitschr. f. Psychologie*, Leipzig, 1930.

[2] *Über das Zustandekommen der Tiefenwahrnehmung mit besonderer Berücksichtigung der Querdisparation.*

graph quoted above. His work has shown that the perception of depth is, even in the adult, not solely dependent on transverse retinal disparity, as is usually assumed.

Like the perceptual world, the imaginal processes are permanently connected with the eidetic sphere. According to the investigations of A. Kobusch,[1] the variable behaviour of images (*Vorstellungen*), which, from the work of G. E. Müller would almost appear to follow no laws and to be chaotic, can to a large extent be explained as follows : according to the inner attitude and the external experimental conditions, images can either be closer to, or further removed from the eidetic sphere. The perceptual world and the world of images and ideas therefore both point to the eidetic sphere. The younger the individual, the closer they are to it. The limiting case would be one in which both exist together as one ' eidetic unity,' which has the characteristics of both worlds. This extreme case is by no means present in all young children. But here and there it is still to be found. We called it the ' unitary type ' (*Einheitstypus*). In the above-mentioned monograph, H. Bamberger[2] describes pronounced cases of that type, in which there often is actual confusion between eidetic phenomena and real objects. Important observations could be made here as to the factors that determine the impression of external reality. The *general* importance of this unitary type is that individuals with a strong eidetic disposition approach this state more or less closely. They therefore all lie on the way to this type.

A consideration of these facts leads us to picture the

---

[1] *Nachweis der Gedächtnisstufen im Vorstellungsleben normaler Erwachsener.*

[2] *Über das Zustandekommen des Wirklichkeitseindrucks der Wahrnehmungswelt.*

development of the perceptual and imaginal world according to the adjoining schema—subject, of course, to limitation or extension :

Perceptions (P) and images (I) differentiate themselves out of their original unity (U). Naturally this does not

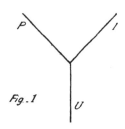

Fig. 1

mean that optical contents will at first arise without a stimulus, that is, be hallucinated We must assume that it is not the endogenous factor in the development of the perceptions, which is primarily responsible for the contents, but forms, and particularly their spatial arrangement. This may be made clearer by a comparison with the doctrines of Kant, which actually receive an empirical foundation through our researches. Kant distinguishes between the matter and the form of experience and thinks that only the latter is a product of the perceptual forms peculiar to consciousness. But we cannot expect to find these differentiating processes in the development of every individual. The theory of types, which has been evolved as a result of eidetic investigations, shows that great differences exist here. Many individuals—the ' disintegrates ' of our typology—receive the structure of their perceptual world as a completed heritage. Those with more plastic, impressionable structures, only develop it during their life, and thus give us evidence of the developmental processes that have been described. It is these individuals who are of special importance to the study of the development of various processes, which at some time will have been completed everywhere. The observations that are made on them can be made the basis of our conceptions about this development in general. In these individuals functions that later are separate, still interpenetrate one another to a high degree and influence each other. That is why we call them 'integrate.' The integrate type is an earlier one from the evolutionary point of view. The younger children are, the more fully do they show this characteristic integration. Integration also dominates the behaviour of primitive peoples.[1]

From what has been said, it is clear that eidetic phenomena are symptoms of more general psychical and physical relationships, which are most obvious in these phenomena, but which also manifest themselves in other spheres. Thus from eidetics we were led more and more into typological investigations. The first studies in this direction were briefly discussed in the first part of this book. They will, I think, be of permanent importance in medical and clinical questions. They have been discussed at length in the monograph of Walther Jaensch, " *Grundzüge einer Physiologie und Klinik der psychophysischen Persönlichkeit* " (Berlin, 1926), which is based on work my brother and I did together.

At that time we started out from eidetic types and, naturally, from pronounced cases. Cases whose symptoms are too one-sided, already begin to border on the pathological, or may even be definitely pathological. Such pronounced cases also have various somatic stigmata according to their type. Thus we obtained insight into various forms of nervousness and their constitutional foundations, particularly in children. The method of capillary microscopy, which was introduced soon after, has meanwhile been extended and

---

[1] Though to a different degree according to their domicile. For, as we shall show later, there is a close correlation between the degree of integration and conditions of light and warmth.

perfected by W. Jaensch [1] and his assistants. As a diagnostic index and therapeutic guide it has had remarkable success. By its means fruitful approaches to the therapy of neuroses and psychoses have been opened up.

Although our doctrine of the basedowoid and tetanoid types (B- and T-types), which was based on the pronounced cases of eidetics, will keep its clinical importance, a general psychology of normality cannot be founded on it. In continually bringing up this criticism, the scientific intuition of psychologists has undoubtedly been correct. Since our typology has repeatedly been subjected to this criticism, I shall discuss this point a little more fully.

E. Kretschmer in particular has been an exponent of the method of gaining insight into normality through its pathological manifestations. I could not take up this standpoint if I did not wish to be subjected to the criticism I had often made against Kretschmer: that, unless artificial relations are established between pathological and normal phenomena, the study of pathological cases can only lead to specialized typologies and cannot embrace the whole of normality. But our starting-point was different to Kretschmer's. He started from definite syndroma, while our work started from phenomena that can be subjected to experimental investigation. We started from pronounced cases, which were easy to recognize and in which fairly rough methods sufficed to bring the various forms to light. The methods merely required being made more accurate to discover the less pronounced cases, or ' latent ' phases of those phenomena. In this way experimental criteria are obtained, to which not only particular individuals, but every individual, can be subjected. Eidetic phenomena

[1] W. Jaensch, *Die Hautkapillarmikroskopie*, Halle, 1929.

can only be examined in eidetic subjects ; but these phenomena are merely a symptom of a general structural personality, which is in evidence far beyond the limited range
of eidetic phenomena.[1]

The barriers that normally exist between sensations and
images seem in eidetic phenomena to have been broken
down, or at any rate diminished in effectiveness. Is there
a similar interpenetration of functions in other respects as
well, not only in eidetic subjects with regard to the eidetic
phenomena, but in other individuals and at other levels ?
In order to decide this, many different experimental methods
were employed. It was mentioned that the investigations
of adaptation, which in the case of children and in many
adults discovered a type of adaptation integrated with the
ideational levels, are still close to eidetic investigation.
Other investigations, which are also still close to eidetic
tests, were made on after-images by means of the intermittence method introduced by Miles in America. This
method gives rise to intensified after-images and enables
one to recognize eidetic components where these do not
appear under direct and simple testing.[2] The intermittence
experiment shows up latent eidetic phenomena. But integration, of which eidetic and latent eidetic phenomena are but
one symptom, is a far wider concept. The integrational
process was gradually traced from the periphery to the
inner psychic life. In perception, all those experiments
give useful criteria, in which the sensory reaction (r) to a
particular complex of stimuli is altered from r to r^1 by the

[1] In what follows, we are referring to eidetic phenomena with a higher
mental component, not to those that are merely intensified after-images.
Only the former are of constitutional importance ; the latter are almost
always pathognomonic. For details, see below.

[2] W. Schmülling, " Aufdeckung latenter eidetischer Phänomene und des
integrierten Typus mit der Intermittenzmethode," *Zeitschr. f. Psychol.*, 105.

circumstances of the experimental setting. Because of the strong mutual interpenetration of functions in the integrate type, the effect of such modifying conditions is very much stronger. As an example we may take the 'co-variation phenomenon.'[1] If three parallel threads are suspended in a plane perpendicularly in front of an observer and one of the side threads is moved forward or backward, the other side thread also appears to change its position, although its co-ordinates on the retina remain the same. The movement of attention, which is called forth by the motion of one thread, influences the apparent position of the one that has not been moved. Only in extreme cases of the integrate type, which are closely related to the 'unitary type,' can the experiment proceed differently. The idea obtained at the beginning of the experiment, that the three threads lie in one plane, influences the subsequent perception so strongly, that the change is not noticed at all. These cases are recognized, first, by the fact that the displacement must be abnormally high in order to be perceived at all ; secondly, by their satisfying the other criteria of the unitary type.

Most of the experiments in perception that are designed to discover the integrate type follow the same principle. A line will very easily alter its apparent length if the subject is pulled by the arms while he is observing. This change in length can take place either spontaneously, or only if the subject projects an imaginary force into the line. This is a criterion for distinguishing between two subtypes of the integrate type, I_1 and I_2.[2] This phenomenon is particularly

[1] F. Kranz, " Experimentall-strukturpsychologische Untersuchungen über die Abhängigkeit der Wahrnehmungswelt vom Persönlichkeitstypus," *Zeitschr. f. Psychol.*, 16. Ergänz. Band, 1930.

[2] E. Jaensch and V. Lucke, " Formen des integrierten Menschentypus," in *Grundformen menschlichen Seins*, by E. Jaensch (und Mitarbeiter), Berlin, 1929.

striking if eidetic images are made of drawings of the Müller-Lyer illusion. Pulling at the arms may lengthen the image by as much as two yards. Such abnormal increases in length when the arms are pulled, are not obtained only in eidetic images ; a basedowoid girl examined by us in the Frankfurt clinic saw a real line lengthening from 5 to 250 cm. In the experiment with Rollett plane parallel converging plates a change in the convergence of the eyes is made and this gives rise to a change in the apparent sizes of objects. Here again, the effect of ' secondary factors,' in this case the degree of convergence, is far greater in the integrate than in the non-integrate (cf. F. Kranz, *op. cit.*).

The Rollett experiment gives rise to a further test used a great deal by us, which leads to the more complex processes of perception. The author had previously shown by means of Hering's haploscope that sensations are intensified when the eyes converge for near vision, so that colour impressions become more intense and more contrasted, while in convergence for distance, depth values are intensified and transverse retinal disparity has a greater effect. ' Psychical assimilation ' is already present in the perception of depth. Experiments on integrates, in whom the secondary conditions —the degree of convergence—have a greater effect, showed that in general, when the eye is focused for distance, a greater degree of ' psychical assimilation ' takes place. The associations that are called up by the objects shown have a greater effect.[1] If the picture that is being shown illustrates some movement, this movement seems to be ' paralysed ' or ' frozen ' when the eyes are strongly

[1] E. Jaensch and E. Neuhaus, " Uber die Persönlichkeitsmerkmale der Übersteigerungsform des integrierten Menschentypus." (*In Grundformen menschlichen Seins.*)

convergent ; but when the eyes are converging for distance vision, the movement is immediately and strongly experienced. Tachistoscopic methods are particularly valuable for investigating the more complete perceptual processes of integrates and non-integrates.[1] Since functions that are usually separate co-operate in the case of the integrate, his perceptions are here dominated above all by large complexes, whilst the non-integrate builds up the whole from its separate parts. In these experiments the ' intuitive ' method of perception of the integrate is in evidence, as against the ' piece-meal,' analytic methods of the non-integrate. This is particularly clearly seen in pronounced cases in the Rollett experiment (Jaensch and Neuhaus, *op. cit.*). One of the chief characteristics of intuition is that the perceiving individual does not stand *next* to the object, but places himself *within* it. This type of apprehension is characteristic of the integrate. One sees over and over again what aversion people of this type have against that form of apprehension in which dividing barriers are set up between the Knower and the Known, preventing immediate union with the object. It is a permanent attitude in which the strong ' coherence ' with the external world, so characteristic of the integrate, finds its expression. Our investigations show that it is a pedagogical necessity to maintain or reconstitute this ' coherence ' with the external world, which is present in childhood.

The development of the theory about integrate and disintegrate types does not invalidate the B and T type theory ; it merely places these two types in a wider context.

---

[1] Oscar Oeser, " Tachistoskopische Leseversuche als Beitrag zur strukturpsychologischen Typenlehre," *Zeitschr. f. Psychol.*, 112, 1930, reprinted in *Studien zur Psychologie menschlicher Typen*, edited by E. R. Jaensch, Leipzig, 1930.

The B and T types are special cases of integrate and disintegrate types, which are distinguished by definite somatic characteristics. Their clinical importance is not in any way affected by limiting their application in normal psychology. In fact the elucidation of their relation to normal types has led to a deeper understanding of them. The investigations of my brother and myself had started from pronounced eidetic cases, which, like all pure types, are not harmonically developed and therefore border on the pathological. From this common basis we tried to find the way to normality. The more extensive our material grew, the more certain we became that, from the point of view of a theory of types, *i.e.* of constitutional dispositions, the B and the T type were not equally valuable, nor could they be looked upon as parallel types in the way in which the older psychology placed the temperaments next to one another. From the results of more recent work, which have been obtained from perfectly normal individuals, it appears that the B type is closer to normal forms, although some of its more pronounced cases border on the pathological. Moreover it is more constitutional and more uniform. The T complex is first of all merely a symptom of a disease or passing indisposition due to endogenous or exogenous disturbing factors. In the latter case, therefore, it is a diseased condition that is not determined by the constitution. The circumstances that bring it about may be quite different in different cases ; they are not at all uniform. Ebbinghaus mentions the common experience that after a sleepless night intensified after-images easily occur. So as a result of accidental and quite different types of injury, individuals who formerly had only the characteristics of the B type may begin to have those of the T type as well. But the converse has never been observed, that individuals with T type stigmata acquired more of the B type accidentally. Wherever eidetic characteristics are retained after the phase of childhood in which they are normal, they are similar to the eidetic characteristics of the B type, that is, they are the highest expression of ' coherence ' with the objective world. But this is only the case where development has been *normal* and unaccompanied by injuries, as in a system of education adapted to the needs of youth. Hence the normal eidetic phenomena of childhood all lie without exception on the way to those of the B type. In the normal case they are never merely intensified after-images.

We have maintained elsewhere that puberty, from the psychical point of view, is above all a period of readjustment as regards the direction of coherence. For coherence with the external objective world there is substituted coherence with the human and mental worlds. If this is kept in mind, the words of the poet F. Werfel can be applied, *mutatis mutandis*, to the normal eidetic phenomena of childhood : " love is nothing more than the capacity for passionately developing the picture of a human being in our inner dark-room." Only instead of " a human being " we must substitute " an object," in order to take into account the tendency of the youthful mind towards the objective universe. The intensified after-images and the symptoms of the T complex could never be characterized by the words of a poet. They are not the expression of a normal tendency of development, but of injurious factors. And in this lies the continued importance for medicine of these phenomena, in our opinion. The psychologist deals in general only with the constitutional type ; the medical man with constitutional type plus disease. There will inevitably be gradual transition stages between the material studied by normal psychology and that studied by the doctor, because of the large number of exogenous and endogenous injurious factors that our civilization brings with it. But, as the progress of our typological researches has clearly shown, both must emphasize different aspects.

It is being shown that two aspects are being more and more differentiated: psychophysical typology and the theory of the constitution of normal personality, and the teaching about the complexes of primary disease now in the process of being developed. The necessity for the latter is evident from the following general considerations. In the epoch that has just passed, medicine was predominantly orientated towards anatomy and its greatest achievement was the development of surgery. It sought the point at which disease attacked the organism in the organ in which the functional disturbance or the anatomical change was observed. To-day it is being realized more and more clearly that these *organic and functional disturbances* observed in individual organs (*e.g.* the stomach), are a secondary effect of different *primary diseases*. They are, to use an analogy from reflexology, the common *end path* in which quite different primary diseases may terminate. We must therefore distinguish between the following : (I) the original cause of the disease ; (II) the complex of primary disease, which is produced in the organism and which may extend into the most diverse functions of the organism ; (III) the end path, that is, the functional or organic change observed in an organ. This end path is common to several 'complexes of primary disease' (II). Various complexes of primary disease, such as changes in the ionic balance, disturbances in the function of the sympathetic or the cerebro-spinal nervous systems, etc., can cause exactly similar changes in the organ, or at any rate changes that are very difficult to distinguish from each other.

The T complex is such a type of primary disease. It is not at all necessary that the complex in question should arise out of a 'T constitution,' to which the individual is specially predisposed. It may be due to the fact that the cause posits a certain *complex* of effects, just as medicines

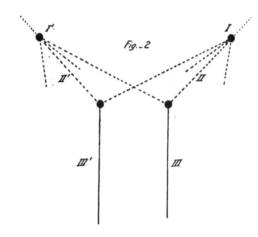

Fig. 2

do. This example of interrelated effects due to medicaments shows very clearly that certain complexes of effects can occur in every organism—though to a different degree in each—without a constitutional disposition for the coming into effect of this complex having to be assumed. The converse is also true : the individual who is now showing this complex would perhaps never have had it, if he had not been exposed to the cause of which the complex is a primary effect. This complex therefore need not be characteristic of his constitution, any more than the complex effects due to a medicament are. From this point of view,

then, as a type of primary disease, the distinction between
the B and the T complex will always be of importance.
In many cases it allows us to decide of what sort the
primary effect is—seen as a primary disease (II)—which is
at the root of the observed functional disturbance in an
organ (III). In particular, as W. Jaensch has shown, it is
often possible to decide whether psycho-therapy will in any
particular case be a true ætiological therapy, or whether the
ætiological therapy should start from the somatic side. In
view of the tendency of psycho-therapy, psycho-analysis
and similar efforts to extend their field without limit, this
will in itself often be of great value. Wherever the T complex is dominant, while the B complex is absent, psycho-
therapy will not be very effective. If the B complex is
more dominant, psycho-genetic somatic disturbances are the
rule, and can therefore be treated psycho-therapeutically.
This phenomenon receives its explanation from the fact that
the B type is a sub-type of the integrate type, in whom
body and mind are far more closely interdependent. Psychical
events can therefore decisively influence somatic events
unfavourably as well as favourably.

This fact, which simply illustrates an exaggeration of
normal behaviour, again confirms the observation made
above, that the B type is of constitutional importance in
quite a different sense to the T type, and that it is far more
closely related to the distinction between ' integrate ' and
' disintegrate.' An individual having the symptoms of the
B complex is integrate ; and the constitution of an integrate
personality is close to that of the B type, whose integration
is over-dominant in certain directions. But it would be
quite wrong to conclude in the same way, that whoever
has the T complex belongs to the disintegrate type and that

the disintegrate must betray himself through having the
T complex. A highly integrate person can acquire the
T complex under the influence of exogenous, particularly
toxic injurious matter.[1] Conversely those disintegrate
individuals, who are very often particularly hale and healthy
and psychically uncomplicated, will in general be free from
the symptoms of the T complex, which always consists of
a definite form of nervous hyperirritability. We have never
observed that a person having the T complex from birth
has acquired the B complex through injurious influences.
The B complex is present *ab initio*. It can be lost, but
cannot be acquired as the result of toxic influences. The
T complex, on the other hand, is never present in a healthy
individual, though it may be acquired by every one, regard-
less of type. This illustrates the fact that the B and T
complexes are rooted in the constitution to different degrees.
It is of pre-eminent theoretical and practical importance
that this should be realized. Many leading medical men
are also of opinion that progress in these subjects depends
to a great extent on the introduction of more accurate
logical and epistemological thought. If B and T complexes
are both thought to be constitutional, one is apt to be
satisfied when one has diagnosed some disturbance as due
to the T complex, or to try a constitutional therapy. But
the recognition of the T complex as a primary disease,
demands first of all that the hidden noxious factors should
be discovered and neutralized.

Types of primary disease may appear to be forms of
personality in the sense of a normal typology. This is due
above all to the fact that such primary diseases may attack

[1] Perhaps this explains the frequency of the B-T complexes in combination.

the *whole* psycho-physical organism. In that case they can only be characterized by taking various functional aspects into account, as in the case of normal types. The lasting importance of W. Jaensch's monograph seems to me to lie in its attempt at defining for the first time such types of primary disease as diseases of the whole psycho-physical constitution. Clinical attempts at classification into ' types ' are probably at bottom attempts at a ' typology of primary diseases,' which are not diseases of special organs, but chiefly of the whole system. These discussions are necessary in the interests of defining the tasks that are germane to normal typology on the one hand, and on the other to the related, but by no means identical, tasks that fall into the clinical sphere.

Another reason for the belief that B and T complexes are of the same order, is that the same methods are often used for investigating both, such as the investigation of after-images. In the case of the B constitution these methods will show up the characteristics of the B complex. In the case of a pure T complex they will (1) show that all the signs of the B complex are absent ; (2) give the T complex characteristics. But (1) and (2) need not be, and normally are not, found together. It is true that (1) is an indication of a definite kind of constitution, for it shows that the constitution of the individual in question is different from the B constitution. But that in itself is no reason for attributing a T constitution to the individual.

The integrate and disintegrate types are true fundamental forms of human existence corresponding, in a sense, to the fundamental forms discovered by biology. A review of the comprehensive material, which had been investigated in many directions by the methods of experimental psychology,

H

' understanding ' (intuitive) psychology, and the physiology
of the senses, showed that the most useful point of view
from which to set up these fundamental types was that of
the *unitas multiplex*, which, according to W. Stern, is the
basic characteristic of the psychic and psycho-physical
personality and, according to F. Kraus, of the physical
personality as well. And indeed true fundamental classes in
the sense discussed above are found, if the various ways in
which this *unitas multiplex* manifests itself are examined.
The psychic functions can either mutually interpenetrate,
or act separately. In the first case we have the type of
integration, in the second, that of disintegration. That these
types are fundamental, is shown by the fact that they are
clearly correlated to easily recognizable main classes of
human existence and to fundamental aspects of all reality.
The chief classes of human existence are special cases of
these fundamental types : the differences between youth
and age, or male and female, or between northern and
southern types as described by race biologists, are all
special cases of the integrate or disintegrate fundamental
types.

That these types are fundamental is also shown by their
conforming to two fundamental distinctions in all real
Being whatever. For the difference between the integrate
and disintegrate structures is no less than the difference
between organic and inorganic types of process, one of the
deepest and most radical distinctions that exists in the
whole of reality. Although the causal interpretations based
by psycho-vitalism on this view are very much open to
criticism and, according to our view and that of many
others, even highly improbable, nevertheless the structural
theory of organic processes evolved by it—as long as it

remains purely descriptive—has a permanent value and may be made the basis of the discussion as to the difference between organic and inorganic types of process. The sharpest distinction that has been drawn, particularly in the works of Driesch, coincides with the distinction between integrate and disintegrate structural types. In some of our earlier publications we compared the disintegrate functional type with a machine, since in both cases the parts are separate and function 'separately.' In his famous experiments on the sea urchin's eggs, Driesch proved that, in contradistinction to a machine, the whole is somehow contained in each of the parts and has to be conceived of as affecting them. Halving the sea urchin's egg does not produce half an organism, as would be expected in the case of a 'growing' machine ; each half still produces a whole, though smaller, organism. But this is precisely the basic characteristic of the integrate type as opposed to the disintegrate.

In the nervous system we find the same difference between organic and inorganic functional types. That is one of the reasons why the controversy between the psychologies of 'wholes' and *Gestalt* psychology on the one hand and the opposed tendencies on the other will not come to rest. Since the most immediate and closest correlate of the psychic personality is in the central nervous system, the fundamental functional differences that exist here will express themselves in the two main types of personality, the integrate and the disintegrate. As has been mentioned before, these are fundamental groups, since other obvious or easily observable fundamental distinctions of human existence can easily be correlated to them. Some of these differences have already been commented upon, others will be immediately clear from the above remarks.

In recent French psychological publications the psychology of Bergson is occasionally described as *psychologie intégrale*. I do not know whether there is any connection between this description and our publications on the integrate type. At any rate the real basis of Bergson's philosophy, as well as the great influence it has had, is the fact that in it the mode of experience of the integrate type receives its clearest, almost classical expression. Bergson himself did not see that his philosophy is determined by his type, any more than other philosophers saw the extent to which their philosophies were determined by their type. Otherwise these systems could not lay claim to universal validity. Bergson justifies the claim that his system presents universal truth by means of a postulate that is not entirely false, but certainly cannot be more than a half-truth. He makes the mode of experiencing reality of the integrate type free from subjectivity, free from all 'anthropo- and typo-morphism,' by saying that the form of apprehension peculiar to this structural type is that which is adequate to organic Being, while conversely inorganic Being is apprehended by forms that are farthest removed from the integrate structure. What is true and what false in this statement can only be analysed adequately on the basis of the theory of categories. But even without careful analysis, it will be clear that this distinction cannot be made in so simple a manner. ' Intuition,' which is so characteristic of the integrate type, can perfectly well operate in mathematics and the exact sciences ; indeed, it must, if productive work is to be achieved. But the integrate type has got an inner relation to art, so that the difference between artistic and inartistic individuals also falls under the fundamental—and far wider—grouping into integrate and disintegrate types. Art, too, is an attempt to revert from the disintegration induced by civilization to organic modes of Being.

The difference between integrate and disintegrate types also includes the distinction between northern and southern types, which has been drawn by race biologists. That integration (in our sense) is ' sun adaptation,' has been proved by investigations of the colour sense of integrates and disintegrates. They again show that integration and disintegration are structural forms, which affect the whole psycho-physical personality, even in its elementary levels.

Cosmical physics distinguishes between ' sunlight ' and ' skylight ' ; the first consists of rays that directly strike the object, *i.e.* penetrate the atmosphere best, the second is the diffuse light due to scattering in the atmosphere. As we go from north to south, it is obvious that the proportion of sunlight in the light falling on the eyes and the organism of living beings will increase, while the proportion of skylight will decrease. In sunlight the longer waves are in the majority, in skylight the shorter. Now according to our latest investigations, increased sensitiveness to red, *i.e.* ' redsightedness,' is in fact sun adaptation ; for it stands in unequivocal correlation to other somatic characteristics that are certainly due to sun adaptation. ' Greensightedness,' on the other hand, is correlated to characteristics that show sun adaptation to be definitely absent. This adaptation to the sun, which is evidenced by ' redsightedness,' is not merely due to a particularly strong pigmentation of the macula, for redsightedness is also present in extramacular regions. But there is an unequivocal correlation between psycho-physical integration and redsightedness, which has been proved to be a sign of sun adaptation. We must therefore conclude that integration is also sun adaptation.

The method used was to make colour equations—red + green =gray, and yellow +blue =gray—on the Maxwell disc, and also Lithium red +Thallium green =Sodium yellow, mixed spectrally. The equations alone do not tell us which component is overvalent and which undervalent. The colour thresholds were therefore also determined, and these gave accurate knowledge as to the relation of the various sensitivities. The investigations of Mr Puhl and Mr Limper were supplementary and were conducted as follows: the former investigated the colour sense of individuals, who from other criteria were known to belong to the integrate type; the latter selected from a heterogeneous number of subjects those cases which were anomalous in one or other respect. Their general constitution was in every case noted or examined. It was found that 'redsightedness' is sun adaptation from the following facts. Among individuals with extreme redsightedness, not a single fair one was found. Persons with dark eyes, dark skin and dark hair were predominantly 'redsighted' and also preferred red, particularly those that were easily browned by the sun. They generally said that they liked walking in the sun, whilst many 'greensighted' persons avoided the sun or even said that the sun " hurt " them. Persons with light-blue eyes, fair skin and hair [1] were without exception green-sighted. If the body was exposed for some time to sunlight, the eyes being carefully shielded, temporary redsightedness was induced. There is also a difference in the colour sense at various seasons: in summer the eye is relatively red-sighted, in winter relatively greensighted. Nearly all extreme redsighted individuals belong to the pronounced integrate type, which is outwardly perceivable in their

---

[1] Red-blonde individuals behave like the dark-haired.

large luminous eyes. Conversely, all more strongly integrate individuals are found to be redsighted. All this shows the correlation between integration and redsightedness, *i.e.* sun adaptation. We cannot as yet generalize, " all redsighted individuals, even in the lesser degrees, are integrate." For among adults who had only a mild degree of redsightedness, we found some in whom the integrate structure was not present in general, nor in the higher mental sphere. But some correlation between dark pigmentation and integrate structure is certainly evident from our investigations as a whole. Even if general integration is not present in all these individuals, they all are found to be integrate with respect to the optical sphere, that is, they show the characteristics of integrates, *e.g.* in adaptation.

If it is possible to discover true fundamental forms in nature, this does not mean that they have to be forced into a few classes. In some forms of typology this danger is undoubtedly present. But the discovery of basic forms means setting up an *open* system within which unlimited progress is possible. This has been the case in biological classification since Cuvier. Cuvier's achievement was the introduction of a method of *subordination*, that is, certain basic forms are distinguished, which are the general structural plan for all subforms subordinated to them, according to the following diagram:

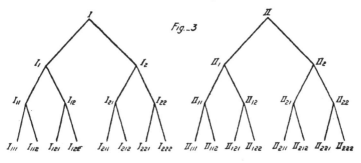

Fig. 3

True basic forms will therefore be traceable in every sub-form and finally in each individual. They are structural plans determining the whole constitution. We have tried to work out such ' basic forms ' according to this schema, which has been of such value in the natural sciences, and the concrete success of the investigations has justified us. The above diagram also shows immediately that the definition of basic forms by no means excludes the infinite variety of types ; they are structural plans for an indefinite number of subforms. But, as the example of science teaches us, investigations must start from the fundamental forms and then proceed to further differentiation. That has been our method ; for we first set up the integrate and disintegrate types and then proceeded to differentiate their various sub-types. The mode of integration may be different, according as it is general or only takes place in a certain direction, or according to the nature of the direction in which integration takes place. Where integration determines an interpenetration of subject and object, the type will be entirely different according as the subjective or the objective component dominates in the integration product. Furthermore, the integration nucleus, *i.e.* the element which in any particular case affects everything else, may be quite different in different cases, etc.

The purely somatic characteristics are sometimes found even in the less pronounced cases, but they are here no longer found every time. But even in these cases, the fundamental characteristic of integration, if it is present at all, will show itself at the higher and the highest levels of the personality. In the type with general integration directed outward, we find a close ' coherence ' of the personality with the outside world, corresponding to the mutual interpenetration in the inner life of those functions through which external reality is presented to the individual. They surrender themselves lovingly to the impressions from outside, as it were. It is not mere chance that we most frequently found integrates, as far as educated adults were concerned, among artistic persons, or persons with general æsthetic interests. The integrate mode of experience is the alphabet of art, and art rests on it. A work of art can portray thoughts, for instance, but in a concretely visualized form, in an ' integration ' of thought and concrete visualization. Perception and feeling, again, are indissolubly integrated in ' empathy.'

Since all functions operate at the same time every cross-section in time will form a unity. In exaggerated cases we have a series of successive cross-sections without the connecting unity of an " ego " running through them. The unitary form of the pronounced integrate type may therefore be characterized as a " cross-sectional unity." The lack of a unity in " longitudinal section," is often evident in a certain weakness of will and sometimes of character, particularly in cases bordering on the pathological.

This is true to a high degree of the synæsthetic (S type), a subform of the integrate type, to which a number of investigations has been devoted. The analysis of the S type brings to light a particularly strong ' autistic ' mode of experience, which gives a picture of the world valid only for the individual himself.

In the integration product, which is the result of the coherence of subject and object, the object dominates in the I_1 type, the subject in the synæsthetic. In place of ' empathy ' (*Einfühlung*) towards persons and objects, the synæsthetic has ' propathy ' (*Zufühlung*). The emotional tone (*Stimmung*) of the I_1 type depends upon external circumstances; that of the synæsthetic is due to his inner circumstances, and he impresses ,his emotional tone on external circumstances and objects. In the relationship of coherence and intimate contact with the outer world, which both the I_1 and the S types have, the receptive attitude is characteristic of the former, whilst the latter is characterized by active productivity. The I_1 type is a 'reception' type; the S type is a 'projection' type. In the latter, inner reflections are so dominant in consciousness, that symbols are often put instead of reality, and the relations of symbols take the place of the relations of external realities. That is why one often gets the impression that the contents of their thinking are loosely connected fragments. They are arbitrarily chosen and are connected by purely inner reflexes. The thoughts of the S type are to those of the I_1 and I_2 types (to be discussed later) as *esprit* is to *Geist*.[1] Such free manipulation of what is given is only possible because all contents and relations are extremely loosely knit, plastic, and easily split apart. This looseness of all contents of inner and outer worlds is often counterbalanced by definite lines of living or thinking being laid down to give a stable organization, which is then projected into the outer world. This particularly applies to geometrical construction or, in general, *esprit de géometrie*, which is introduced by the mind as a means to stable organization. Typical French thought has all the valuable and the shady sides of synæsthetic structure.

The I_1 type is *unconditionally* open to reality, the S type

[1] The sense in which these two words are used here may perhaps be made a little clearer by the following : A joke that has *esprit* depends for its effect on two absolutely disparate facts being brought together by some brilliant mental *salto mortale* ; if it has *Geist* it depends more on actual subtle logical connections between the two facts or aspects. [Trans.]

only *conditionally*, only for that on which the beam of light from within has fallen. Because of this particular form of coherence with reality, the S type is always liable to split off from reality ; and being open to influences from without may easily change over to estrangement from reality.[1]

Investigations in the field of literature by Erika von Siebold and others, have shown that synæsthetic phenomena occur most often in French, least in English, and to a moderate degree in German literature. The synæsthetic is a very primordial type, which is widely found in childhood (H. Freiling). The unity that in the S type extends over and connects the different sensory fields in the form of inner reflexes, is probably the *sensorium commune* sought by Herder. According to his teaching it is the basis of the

---

[1] In this way we may explain the close connection between the synæsthetic and the ' schizoid ' type of Kretschmer. But the so-called ' schizoids ' are by no means a uniform group. It contains synæsthetics, disintegrates, the purely inwardly integrated type, and the I_2 type. Kretschmer's ' pykniks ' are a particular case of the I_1 type. The pronounced ' schizoids ' first described by Kretschmer in " Physique and Character " correspond to our synæsthetics. Only in the later experimental work of Kretschmer and Kroh do the disintegrates, pure inward integrates, and individuals of the I_2 type appear among their ' schizoids.' This lack of uniformity of the so-called ' schizoid group ' is the reason for the results of various investigators sometimes flatly contradicting each other (Enke and Heising—Kroh and his pupils). Moreover, since the most pronounced ' schizoids ' first described by Kretschmer correspond to our S type, and the ' pykniks ' to a subform of the integrate (I_1) type, I_1 and S types should be at opposite poles. But that is in no way confirmed by our investigations of these types (Jaensch—Neuhaus, Jaensch—Lucke and Jaensch—Ingeburg Meier in *Grundformen menschlichen Seins*). There is no contradiction between S and I_1 types. They are both co-ordinated under the wider group of the integrate type. Hence there is a gradual transition between the I_1 and the S type, according to the increasing importance of the subjective component in the coherence relation and the increasing liability to ' splitting off.' This is clearly shown by the fact that in the investigations of J.—Ingeburg Meier the observations made by J.—Neuhaus and J.—Lucke had to some extent to be repeated. In order to emphasize this fact, we have purposely not deleted these repetitions.

The integrate and disintegrate types are true polar opposites.

development of language, among other things, since it is the first and primary mediator between the described perceptual complexes of objects and the descriptive sound complexes of language. The S type also tends to introduce geometrical symbols for reality. Indeed, he tends to replace reality by these symbols, a process that was of great importance in the beginning and development of modern science, when science was chiefly based on geometry.[1]

It is not possible to touch upon the most important subforms of the integrate and disintegrate types in such a short summary as this. The I_2 type, which is integrate at certain times and under special conditions, shows the transition from the transient moment-to-moment unity (*Querschnitteinheit*, ' cross-sectional unity ') to the more permanent unity (*Längsschnitteinheit*, ' unity in longitudinal section '). The individual who is *generally* integrate, is always in intimate contact and ' coherence ' with the external world ; the *conditionally* integrate I_2 type only when the outer world corresponds to certain fixed complexes of his inner life, in particular, his ideals.[2] These complexes are deeply rooted in his emotions and sentiments. They are not only apprehended by his reason, and are therefore not limited to the superficial layers of personality. We have likened the consciousness of the generally integrate I_1 type to an empty space, which receives its contents from the environment. But in the I_2 type definite conceptual and emotional complexes, ideas and ideals, form a nucleus

---

[1] The predominant and one-sided influence of the point of view of the S type on our systems of scientific thought is discussed in " Über den latenten Cartesianismus der Modernen Wissenschaft," 16. *Ergänz. Bd.*, *Zeitschr. f. Psychol.*, 1930.

[2] In the S type even these firmly and deeply-rooted complexes are lacking.

for the personality which is permanent in time, a 'unity in longitudinal section.' The I_2 type is in 'coherence' with the external world only through these. But in it, too, the fundamental structure runs through all levels. Hence the I_2 type can be experimentally discovered, since in the most elementary perceptual processes similar aspects to those of the higher mental life are found.

As the outward integration and connection decrease, to be replaced more and more by inner integration of firmly rooted complexes, the characteristics of the pure, *inwardly* integrate type begin to appear. It is the polar opposite of the outwardly integrate type. His values are character and a stable line of life, corresponding to the inward integration and the firm, sometimes even rigid complexes of his inner life. The lower degree of 'coherence' is also recognizable by experimental criteria. Eidetic phenomena presuppose a high degree of coherence with the external world; visual images, which are connected with eidetic images by gradual transition stages, at any rate presuppose a medium degree of coherence. But in the type we are considering visual imagery is almost completely absent. In its stead we find motor and dynamic contents. Even at elementary levels these express a more practical and active attitude to outside reality, than is the case in the 'coherence' relationships of the outwardly integrate type.

The general philosophic import of these investigations seems to us to be the following: the question of *a priori* categories, which runs through the whole history of epistemological problems, is placed on a new basis; they make possible a more logically consistent development of empiricism; and they promote mutual tolerance, in epistemological systems as well as in the whole communal life of man.

The theory of perception that is based on eidetic investigations shows that in our inner world of ideas (*Vorstellungswelt*), an inner, *a priori* factor, is intimately concerned in the development of the perceptual world. Although in his work on Kant M. Heidegger [1] does not mention the theory of perception and the epistemology based on eidetics, this latest and most penetrating interpretation of Kantian philosophy shows us that Kant was already aiming at these results of modern empirical and philosophical anthropology, and that some of its fundamental results have been preestablished by his profound intuition. For, from the way in which he describes it, the *Einbildungskraft* that he conceives as the basis of our form of spatial perception, is the same as the eidetic faculty ; and when he describes it as the common root of " the two branches, sensibility and reason," he is intuitively perceiving that the worlds of sensation and of ideas have a common origin in the " primary eidetic unity."

Our investigations show that, like the perceptual world, our world of thought and knowledge is decisively determined by the structure of our consciousness. The kind of structure differs in the various fundamental types. The systems of knowledge of the different sciences are also based to a large extent on the different type of mind-structure operating in them. Different categories correspond to each. Each structure of consciousness separates out different aspects of reality, by reproducing certain categories of reality through the medium of categories of consciousness that are related to them. Those categories of reality, in which corresponding categories of consciousness are not present, remain unapproachable and are apprehended through

[1] *Kant und das Problem der Metaphysik*, Bonn, 1929.

different structures. The danger of one-sidedness, sub-jectivity and error in the fundamental questions of know-ledge, is chiefly due to the fact that every structure of consciousness claims unlimited validity ; but in truth each makes very wide negative abstractions of reality. We can, therefore, only penetrate reality and approach the ideal of ' pure experience ' by successively taking up the standpoints of different mental structures. The typological basis of epistemology thus includes the principle of tolerance. Bitter controversies, such as those that have been fought in Germany about the relation of scientific and historical method, will no longer be possible.

In the interests of objectivity and the progress of know-ledge we must raise the question whether the different structures have had an equal influence in building up our systems of knowledge. An investigation of this question shows that in the system of science the constructive, ration-alistic, Cartesian structure has been over-emphasized, as is to be expected from historical considerations.[1] This is the structure that corresponds to the ' synæsthetic ' subform of the integrate type. Empiricism, and the standpoint of empirical reality, which is in some respects alien to the Cartesian structure, have not yet received due recognition. This can be shown to be true not only in philosophy, but in the special sciences as well, even in the most exact. We believe that we are not far wrong in attributing the empirical attitude above all to English and German thought. But typology does not demand a new domination ; it demands equality and the equal consideration of all important mental structures. Every structure has its value for humanity.

[1] Cf. last chapter, 16. *Ergänz. Bd., Zeitschr. f. Psychol.,* 1930.

This is also evident in the investigations of religious [1] and æsthetic [2] experience, which assume different forms in different structures, but which always include a *variety* of values. Different peoples, too, are of different structures, not merely because of different descent and historical development, but also because environment may determine the type, as has been shown by our researches on the influence of light.

[1] E. Jaensch, " Psychologische Typenforschung und Wertphilosophie, mit besonderer Rücksicht auf die Fragen der Religionspsychologie." 10. *Kongress für experim. Psychol.*, Bonn, 1927.

E. Jaensch, " Psychological and psychophysical investigations of types in their relation to the Psychology of Religion," in *Feelings and Emotions, the Wittenberg Symposium*, Worcester, Mass., 1928.

[2] *Studien zur psychologischen Ästhetik und Kunstpsychologie*, edited by E. Jaensch, Langensalza, 1929.

APPENDIX

EIDETICS, THE DEVELOPMENT OF PERCEPTION, AND THE BASES OF OUR CONCEPTION OF REALITY. A DISCUSSION OF SOME CONTROVERSIES

SOME psychologists still look upon eidetic phenomena as an interesting special study, as a characteristic of a few individuals, but not as a matter of supreme importance to psychology and epistemology in *general*. But if that were so, we should not have devoted so much time and labour to eidetics, since we have from the very beginning always turned to those questions of general importance, which are awaiting solution in the fields of psychology and philosophy. We have not made eidetics the centre of our investigations for so long because of a chance discovery, but because we soon realized its importance for general psychology and several of its neighbouring sciences.

Three main arguments are usually advanced for not attributing *general* importance to eidetics.

(1) We attribute the importance of this study to the fact that eidetic phenomena play such a large part in the development of perceptions. Since this takes place during *early* childhood, the phenomena should be most frequent at this age, if they are to have the function that we attribute to them. Some psychologists, however, have asserted that eidetic phenomena are at a maximum in the period preceding *puberty*.

I

(2) Manifest eidetic phenomena are not found in *every* child. But if they are to play a fundamental part in building up the perceptual world, it is argued that they ought to be present in every, or nearly every, individual. We have found characteristics that are present in every one, and have called them 'latent eidetic phenomena.' This term has been assailed by various theoretical and dialectic arguments.

(3) Some writers seem to admit 'latent eidetic phenomena,' but deny that they have anything to do with the development of perceptions.

Now these arguments are nearly always put in a purely theoretical form. But we are not dealing with theoretical questions here at all ; they are purely questions of *fact*, and I can only ask my opponents over and again to test these *facts* for themselves. They have been verified by us and by others so often, from such diverse points of view, that I am quite content to take up a waiting attitude towards their attacks. But since we had occasion to touch on these questions in the body of the work, I shall take this opportunity of discussing them again here.

(1) Our own work and the quite independent work of Roessler [1] has shown the supposition, that eidetic phenomena are a peculiar characteristic of pre-puberty, to be quite untenable. Roessler found, in agreement with us, that eidetic phenomena become increasingly prevalent as earlier ages are investigated.

(2) *All* children have not got eidetic images. That is

---

[1] F. Roessler, " Verbreitung und Erscheinungsweise subjektiver optischer Anschauungsbilder bei Knaben und Mädchen im Alter von 6-10 Jahren,' *Beihefte der Zeitschr. für angew. Psychol.*, 43, 1928.

well known to us, and we have never asserted the contrary. But this does not in the least diminish the general importance of eidetic images, which lies in the fact that they are the clearest *indicators* for certain structures appearing during specific phases of childhood and sometimes remaining permanently. These structures are found to be universally distributed, or nearly so, at the respective ages, and they go beyond the sphere of eidetic images. They are the previously mentioned 'hemieidetic' characteristics of perceptual processes. The perceptions of children and of adults who are of a permanently youthful type, are actually 'half' eidetic. J. Gross, for instance, found that after-images with a hemieidetic character, *i.e.* with similar characteristics to eidetic images, are extremely common among children. Various tests also showed that hemi-eidetic spatial perceptions are extremely common in childhood.[1] Like Gross, H. Ruschmann and Ella Mayer carried out their investigations of the perceptual processes of children on a normal material, which had not been specially sifted for eidetic phenomena.[2] They, too, found that in children the perception of depth has a hemieidetic character. Just as in the case of eidetic subjects, peripheral factors dependent on stimuli, in particular transverse retinal disparity, have a relatively small effect in children, as compared with endogenous 'hemieidetic' factors, which are projected into the perceptions. How deeply these processes, or their later 'precipitates,' affect even the perceptual processes of adults, has been shown by F. Simon.[2] Here it is shown that transverse disparity has by no means the exclusive deter-

[1] J. Gross, in *Studien zur Psychologie menschlicher Typen*, by E. Jaensch u. Mitarbeiter, Leipzig, 1930.

[2] H. Ruschmann, Ella Mayer, and F. Simon, in 16. *Erg.-Bd., Zeitschr. f. Psychol.*, 1929.

mining power, as opposed to central ' projected ' factors, as has hitherto always been assumed.

The above-mentioned phenomena are what we have called ' latent eidetics.' This term has been much criticized. The name is of minor importance and I do not attach any great value to it. But the facts which it characterizes remain ; and they will be accepted, even if slowly. The question can obviously not be decided by theoretical speculations, which so far has been the only form in which criticism has been couched, since the term does not express theoretical postulates, but purely empirical facts. I can only ask those, who deny the existence of latent eidetic phenomena in the sense in which I use the term, to carry out experiments on the perceptions of children and of adults who are of a permanent youthful type, *i.e.*, adults who are strongly integrated outwards. They will then be able to verify that the perceptual processes of children and integrate adults differ from those of average adults, in that their behaviour approximates to that of eidetic images. The perceptual processes receive an *eidetic component*, while the peripheral component, the determining power of external stimuli, is diminished. Although, as I said before, the term ' *latent* eidetic phenomena ' is of minor importance, I nevertheless think it correctly expresses the facts of ' hemieidetic ' phenomena, which contain a strong eidetic component.

That these phenomena should be termed ' latently eidetic,' is also made apparent by the following observation, which we have made again and again. In our work we have distinguished between eidetic manifestations of different strength and, therefore, between subjects who have them in more or less pronounced forms. Consider such a group of different eidetic subjects and also a group of non-eidetic subjects. We shall denote the eidetic phenomena by E, the perceptions of the same person by P. When E and P stand next to each other (E—P), they refer to the same individual. Perceptual processes that have an eidetic component are denoted by P_E. Numerical indices are introduced to express the degree of intensity of the eidetic phenomena, or of their component in the perceptual processes. The higher the index number, the intenser are the eidetic manifestations, or their component in perceptual processes. O means that eidetic phenomena or eidetic components are no longer demonstrable. If we now express our observations schematically, they always give the following correlations :

(1)	E_3	— PE_V
(2)	E_2	— PE_{IV}
(3)	E_1	— PE_{III}
(4)	E_0	— PE_{II}
(5)	E_0	— PE_I
(6)	E_0	— PE_0

Expressed in words : the particular component contained in the perceptions of children and strongly integrate adults does not merely manifest itself as " latent eidetic " because it makes the appearance and the laws of P approximate to those of E, but also because this component is correlated with eidetic phenomena. The most pronounced eidetic individuals also have this component in its strongest form, and the more manifest the eidetic phenomena are, the more effective it is. Nevertheless the above table does not show the correlation completely. In the case of non-eidetic subjects (4–6), we naturally cannot speak of degrees of eidetic faculty, although eidetic components can be traced in their perceptions. The scale of correlation will be complete, if we investigate in addition not only these symptoms, but the whole type, the degree of integration of the individual. It then becomes clear that eidetic phenomena and perceptual processes with an eidetic component are both correlated to this degree of integration ; both are its common expression.

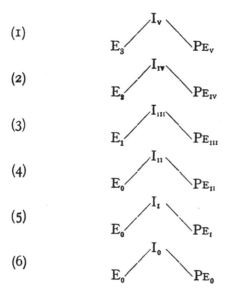

(1) $\quad E_3 \diagup^{I_v}\diagdown PE_v$

(2) $\quad E_2 \diagup^{I_{IV}}\diagdown PE_{IV}$

(3) $\quad E_1 \diagup^{I_{III}}\diagdown PE_{III}$

(4) $\quad E_0 \diagup^{I_{II}}\diagdown PE_{II}$

(5) $\quad E_0 \diagup^{I_I}\diagdown PE_I$

(6) $\quad E_0 \diagup^{I_0}\diagdown PE_0$

The correlation of E and P thus remains incomplete, if we only take these two into consideration. It is completed by considering their common correlation to a third factor. This common correlation to a third, basic, factor, is the true reason for the correlation that was first discovered. The method followed here, or rather, the method which arose naturally during the progress of our investigations, is one of the most common methods for establishing the completeness of a correlation, which at first sight seems to be incomplete.

Those are the facts on which the concept of 'latent eidetic' phenomena has been based. Strictly speaking, even this does not represent all of the facts. They will be fully represented if the above table is repeated once more and P replaced by I =images (*Vorstellungen*). Like perceptions, ordinary memory images can have an eidetic component, without becoming eidetic images, as their behaviour in certain experimental situations has shown.[1] The above correlation for the P's is, however, the more important. The concept 'latent eidetics' is based mainly on this correlation, since the investigation of the P's and their correlations can be carried out far more easily and exactly than that of the I's and their correlations.

(3) The investigation of 'hemieidetic perceptual processes' leaves no doubt that they are of the utmost importance in the development of perceptions. All those factors, which, even in the more stable perceptions of average adults, are of importance for localization (optical-dynamic processes, eye movements, variations in attention, antagonistic processes, assimilation phenomena, etc.), have an incomparably greater effect here. Primordial, 'hemieidetic' perception is to a high degree plastic and modifiable by these localizing factors. This shows itself in the higher degree of illusion produced by these factors (Horopter-deviation, co-variation phenomenon, etc.). A gradual increase of rigidity takes place. It is possible to show that a formation of 'petrifactions' and 'precipitates' of these factors concerned in the development of localization takes place, wherever they are still fully active and the material is plastic. These petrifactions are taken into the whole process by which the perceptions become 'rigid' and are preserved in them.

[1] Cf. A. Kobusch, in 16. *Erg.-Bd.*, *Zeitschr. f. Psychol.*, 1930.

The import of eidetics and latent eidetics for the development of perceptions can also be made clear from a consideration of the generally accepted views of empiricism as to the origin of spatial perception. Although Helmholtz's attempt to base his theory of spatial perception solely on experience has been criticized, it is nevertheless admitted that imaginal and experiential residues play an important part. But this is obviously not true of *all* such residues. I can place two metre sticks at very different distances from my eyes; but although I know perfectly well that they are equal, my knowledge will not make me *see* them as equal. Imaginal and ideational residues must therefore be present in a certain form, if they are to play a part in the building up of the perceptual world. An image based only on knowledge is not sufficient. Helmholtz's theory of perception shows a gap here. It is filled by eidetics, which shows that there are residues of images and experiences capable of being parts of the structure of perceptions, because they are concrete (*anschaulich*) and not, like many contents of knowledge, purely abstract (*unanschaulich*). From this point of view, too, the importance of ' latent ' and ' hemieidetic ' phenomena is clear ; for an eidetic disposition, which is not developed strongly enough to give rise to manifest eidetic phenomena, can nevertheless be intimately concerned in the development of perceptions. Our eidetic investigations have shown again and again that the appearance of eidetic phenomena is considerably facilitated if certain conditions obtain in the outside world, which form a point of contact for them, as it were. This will be the case where, for instance, the data of perceptions to some extent already include the contents of these phenomena, so that they do not arise out of nothing, but fill in a given frame, like a painting arises out of the preliminary sketch.

In our own investigations we followed the progress of many young individuals through a number of years and noted the changes that took place. In this way we came to the conclusion that the perceptions pass through a building-up process. That this is so, has also been sufficiently proved by the older empiricism, e.g. in its observations of people who were born blind and received sight later, and of people who were operated upon and had to learn to see and to localize. The development of perceptions passes through several phases. In each phase the perceptual world is as yet incomplete and is related to the final form as a rich, completed drawing is to the original sketch. At each stage preceding the final completion, the contents of perception offer certain sketches and outlines, which can make even a weak eidetic disposition active. This disposition will then fill in the details with its products, however far removed these may be from manifest eidetic phenomena. Detailed experimental investigations have shown us that all eidetic elements are easily fitted into the external world and, from the point of view of the observer, become a part of it, if they find 'points of contact' in the above-mentioned sense, a frame they can fill or a sketch they can complete.[1]

If our experiments on perception are repeated elsewhere, it must always be remembered that different results are to be expected in different countries, even in different parts of the same country. But this does not mean that chaos takes the place of law: these differences are themselves subject to laws and their direction can be accurately foretold.

[1] Cf. H. Bamberger, in 16. *Erg.-Bd., Zeitschr. f. Psychol.*, 1930.

Like the degree of integration of the psychophysical personality, they are essentially a function of light and temperature. We have always emphasized that the plastic stages of perceptual processes, in which we can follow their development and see their determining factors operating, are no longer observable in each individual. Some individuals inherit a more or less fully developed perceptual world. To what extent this is true, depends on the degree of outward integration, which, in turn, is largely a function of light and temperature. How extremely plastic the psychophysical organism is, can be seen from the fact that relatively small changes in the geo-physical environment produce enormous variations.

The conditions in France and Germany can be compared on the basis of our investigations on the development of perception, which have been carried out in both countries. The plastic, modifiable stage of perceptual processes, in which the factors concerned in the building-up process can be observed, are incomparably more in evidence in France, especially in the south of France. It is found at an age long after it has disappeared in Germany. Experimental data are not as yet available for Italy and Spain. But from general considerations and from observations as to the presence of pronounced outwardly integrated individuals, we may expect even greater differences than between Germany and the south of France. It is to be expected in Spain, particularly.

From what has been said about the relation between the structure of perception and fundamental types, and the distribution of fundamental types, it may be almost certainly predicted that in England and North America the type that is outwardly more disintegrate will predominate. Conditions there will be even further removed from those in France than they are in Germany, so that Germany, from the typological point of view as well as regards the structure of perceptions, will be midway between France on the one hand, and England and North America on the other. In these two regions the 'hemieidetic' character of perceptions will be far less pronounced, and we may expect to find a gradual diminution, as well as an accelerated development, of their plastic phases. There will be a much more definite correspondence of perceptions to external stimuli, or, what amounts to the same, a stronger determining force in external stimuli.

In emphasizing the relation between geo-physical factors, the degree of integration, and the structure of perceptions, we are basing our conclusions on experimental results. These correlations, which are obvious from quite general observations, have also been quite definitely established by experimental investigations of individual differences in the colour sense. These individual differences in the colour sense show a definite correlation on the one hand to the conditions of integration, on the other—no less definitely— to those of light. Although we are following these empirical findings, we do not wish to deny that the cultural environment also has an influence in forming the individual, even his elementary, psychophysical levels. It is, for instance, our view — which we can support by good reasons — that French culture leads in the same direction as the original constitution of the mass of the people. The system of education, which is designed on Cartesian lines of thought, is concerned above all with producing clear, easily impressed *ideas*, while less emphasis is laid on an objectivity that tries to follow the objective data of reality.[1]   In this way a form of experience is induced which favours the subjective component in the relation of ' coherence ' between subject and object, while objective reality has a smaller determining power in forming the outlook on the world.

Between the spirit of the individual and the spirit of civilization there is always a mutual relationship.   This will be of such a form—and in France it certainly is—that the cultural spirit grows out of the spiritual life of individuals, so sharing its nature ; and because of this agreement between the two, it is able to react on and *re-enforce* the structural nature of the individual spirit.

---

[1] Cf. our " Erläuterungen zur Lehre von den menschlichen Grundformen mit besonderer Rücksicht auf die Fragen der Völkerpsychologie," in *Über den Aufbau der Wahrnehmungswelt und die Grundlagen der menschlichen Erkenntnis*, Part II (appearing shortly).

INDEX OF NAMES

OESER, OSCAR, 81, 98

PETERSEN, P., 14, 42
Plato, 49
Poincaré, H., 44
Puhl, 110
Purkinje, 15, 87

RÉVÉSZ, G., 90
Rickert, 35, 53, 55
Riehl, A., 20, 78
Rollett, 97
Rössler, 83 f., 122
Rousseau, J. J., 42
Ruschmann, H., 123

SCHMITZ, KAROLINE, 83
Schmülling, W., 95
Scholl, 69
Schuppe, W., 43
Schwab, G., 8, 17, 18
Siebold, E. v., 115
Simon, F., 90, 123
Sommer, R., 47

Spinoza, 42
Spranger, E., 26, 36, 75, 76
Stern, W., 106
Störring, G., 72
Stresemann, 82

THURNWALD, R., 23
Tschermak, A. v., 35

VERWORN, M., 34

WECHSSLER, 22
Weiss, E., 63
Wenckebach, F., 44
Werfel, F., 100
Wilmanns, 66
Windelband, 53, 55
Wittneben, W., 61
Wundt, Max, 42
Wundt, W., 14, 42

ZEMAN, H., 18
Zillig, M., 18, 25

INDEX OF SUBJECTS